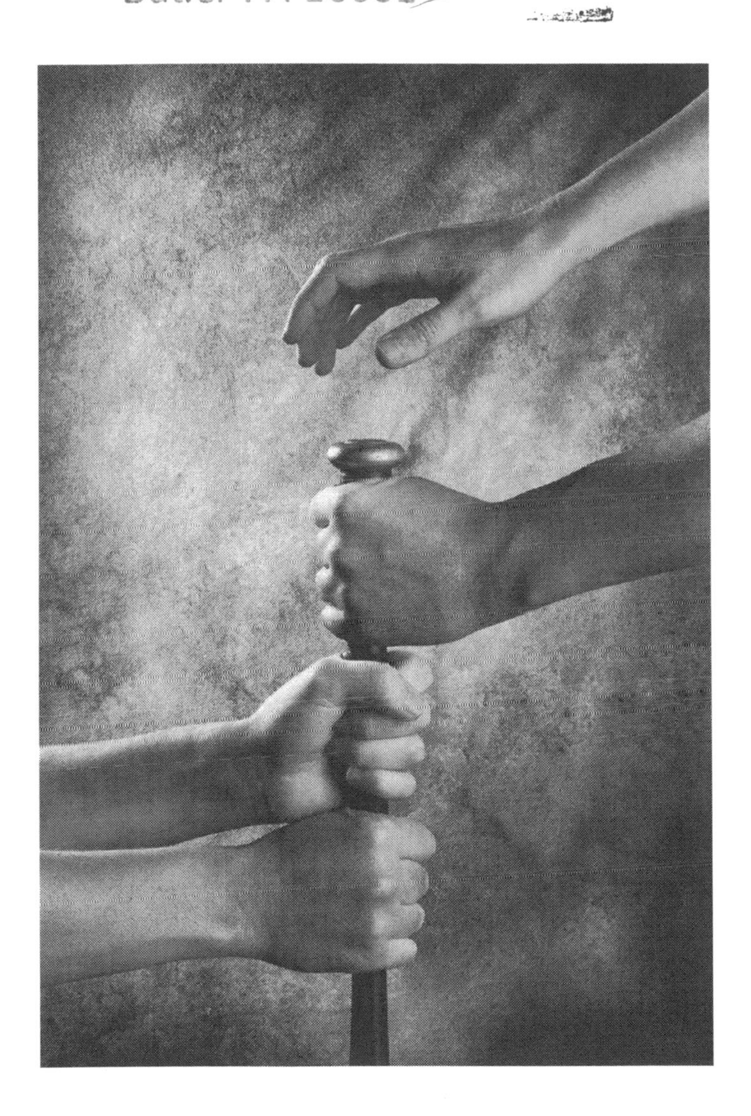

Conquering Lou Gehrig's Disease

The ALS Diet

Hannah Yoseph, MD

ISBN-13: 978-0-9854490-3-2

Published 2012 by James and Hannah Yoseph
jandhyoseph@yahoo.com

Printed in the USA

Galaxy photos by NASA
VCell images of ATP Synthase by Virtual Cell Collection
http://vcell.ndsu.nodak.edu

The information given in this book is solely for educational purposes and is not intended as medical advice.

To order additional copies, please contact the Yosephs at:
jandhyoseph@yahoo.com

First Edition, 2012

Table of Contents

Preface

I was blessed to have a friend, mentor and teacher who was a spiritual man of a different order. One day we were discussing prayer. Suddenly he said, "Don't ever pray for me to live." I was stunned. I loved and honored him enough to not question his request. I simply promised.

He was a pilot. He loved to fly. At the time he spoke that injunction he was sick and tired of living without any quality life. He was tired of living without flying.

For over ten years, I, too, have wrestled with a slow, health sapping enemy. I know what it's like to give up on prayer and all remedy that is founded in hope. Hope came, but it wasn't from my friends, fellow physicians or even my family. It came from Wisdom from within.

If you have been diagnosed with ALS, you are confronting the horror of a lifetime. This is my promise to you. This book is true "do no harm" medicine. It is about health restoration. It is founded in knowledge and wisdom. It is about real answers based upon proven and applied science to restore and maintain cellular health.

The cause for ALS has been known for many years. It is well documented in this book. The logical and simple mode of remedy follows proven cause.

Life is wired to be. My hope for you is that you find health, peace and quality life.

Introduction

Three years ago I had one of those blazing eureka moments. Hannah and I were discussing her then new book on diet and weight loss. I jumped from my chair and started pacing the floor and shouted, "Hannah, you've got it. You've got it all!"

As a carpenter I know how to assemble a myriad of pieces to make a recognizable whole. In my years in the trade I had found that the most direct way to build anything was to first see it finished. Then the process became one of removing obstacles, the details and chasing the materials. The steps became irrelevant. The goal was what mattered. It was my gift, a birthright if you will.

On complicated work, I would sit on a job site, sometimes for days, until I could see the project completed with every piece in place before I would begin.

I finished many projects.

Hannah has assembled a myriad of pieces. She spent years in independent study putting them together one piece at a time. It is a remarkable gift. Good scientific study exists all over the world: cancer research, MS research, ALS research, diabetes research and many more. Her gift is to consolidate it, to connect the dots and make a recognizable whole.

When Einstein published "The Theory of Relativity," someone wrote that only two or three people in the world could even comprehend what he was saying. Such is the depth of Hannah's understanding of cellular health.

I predict that one day Hannah will be considered the mother of cellular health – a breakthrough in modern medicine. In the meantime it will be left to common people like me and you to see the beautiful logic and reasoning it takes to bring together such a massive body of evidence.

Well done my darling; well done!

James B. Yoseph
May 8, 2012

PART ONE: CLEAN UP YOUR POOL

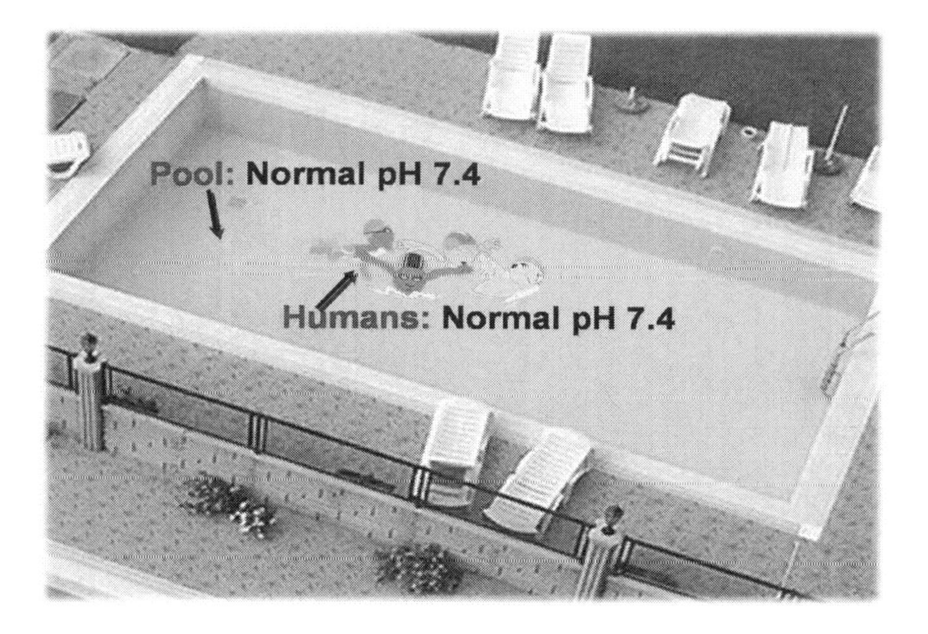

Chapter 1: Food as Medicine

"Let food be your medicine and medicine be your food."
-Hippocrates

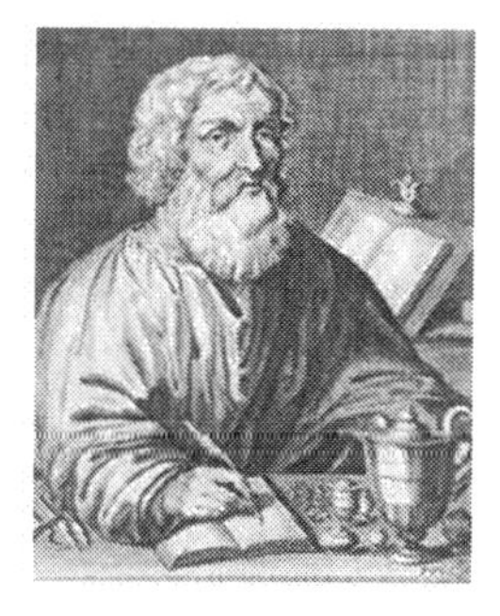

What could Hippocrates have possibly been thinking? Not only is his famous quote redundant; he seems to be saying the same thing twice!

If food is our medicine, then *of course* medicine is our food! Surely there must be something else that Hippocrates meant, only missed on first read.

Hippocrates' advice can be deciphered by substituting his logic with similar constructs such as: "Let soap be your cleaner and cleaner be your soap." Or, "Let the sun be the warmth on your face, and the warmth on your face be the sun."

Aha! Now we can more clearly see how he was *not* being redundant. Soap cleans the skin and the sun warms one's face. But one can wash with baking soda instead of soap and one's face can be warmed with a fire instead of the sun.

Food is medicine. This statement is absolute because it is only food, and nothing else, that can preserve health. But, should we eat the wrong food and lose our health, we can use chemicals as medicine instead of food. Hippocrates said, "Don't; ***let medicine be your food***."

Here is what the father of medicine was saying: "Choose food when you are healthy as if it is your medicine and ***if you lose your health, think twice about what you are eating***." This wise saying is more than good food for thought; it's good medicine! It is the foundation of the wisdom in this book.

Food – and drink – are medicine. In Hippocrates' day, water drawn from wells was the mainstay of drink. Today we drink all kinds of strange concoctions, and usually don't think twice about how it might – *and does* – affect our health.

The ALS diet is about the power of hydrogen in both water and food.

The tiniest of atoms on earth, hydrogen, is what lights up the night sky and is the "stuff" of spinning galaxies. Spinning hydrogen in your cells is also the stuff that energizes you – when in balance and working optimally!

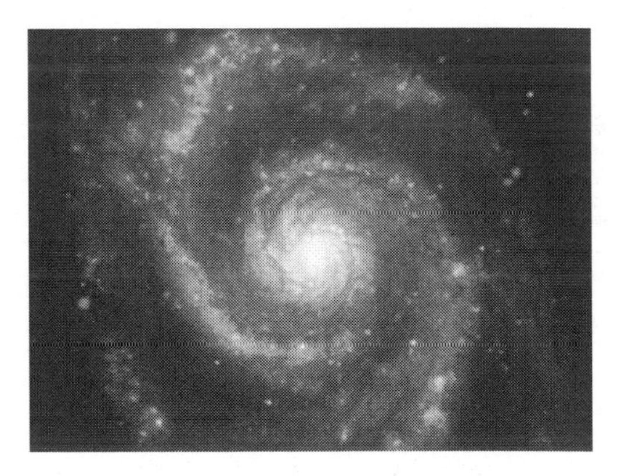

Every human cell is a microscopic universe of spinning hydrogen atoms constantly making and recycling billions of molecules of energy. When you know how to harness the power of hydrogen in both water and food and convert it into maximum energy, you will have the most powerful tool to conquer ALS and stay healthy and fit for life.

Bottom Line: Harnessing the power of hydrogen in food and water is real medicine.

Chapter 2: Health Restoration

"The doctor of the future will give no medicine, but will interest his patients in the cause and prevention of disease."
-Thomas Edison

If any cell is low on energy normally made from nutritious food, it simply cannot perform its normal function any more than a car can run well without clean gas.

With few exceptions, chronic inflammatory neurodegenerative diseases like ALS are due to chronic infection, circulating toxins and acidity exacerbated by nutritional deficiency.

On the surface, ALS appears to be a disorder of autoimmunity. If it was that simple, then suppressing the immune system should restore health. But when ALS flares up, suppressing it with steroids only temporarily make everything feel better; in a matter of time, another flare-up rears its ugly head. The experience of most ALS sufferers is that of a merry-go-round of disease and remission, recovery and flare-up. "Cure" is a four-letter-word.

The practice of traditional medicine accounts for only *symptoms* of deficiency in organs and tissues; treatments are rarely focused at the cellular level. In fact, many diseases are simply terms that, often in Greek, describe the obvious symptoms of a deficient condition that begins in cells.

For example, the diagnosis of a red nose is "rosacea" which means "red." Dry skin is "eczema" which means "to boil over" because the skin sometimes "weeps." Memory or cognition loss is "dementia" which means "without mentation." A sore and swollen joint is called "arthritis" which means "inflamed joint." The diagnosis for degenerating joints is "degenerative joint disease." Excess fat from metabolic insufficiency is called "obesity" which means "too much body fat." A spinal disc that slips out of place (or herniates) due to a deteriorating spine is "herniated disc disease."

"Amyotrophic Lateral Sclerosis" is no exception. It means "muscle wasting many lateral scars".

Endless is the list of scary-sounding names that offer suffering people a modicum of comfort, because at least their pain has a scary name! With a name for a disease, one can also find a support group or at best empathy from friends and family because one's suffering has been validated by a god-like figure.

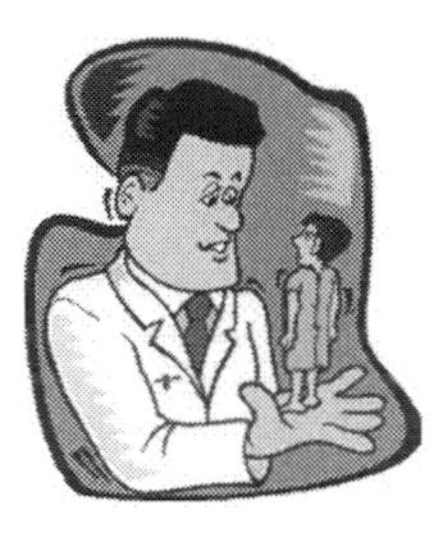

More often than not, the diagnosis for a chronic disease like ALS only describes symptoms and not cause. Drugs, more often than not, likewise treat symptoms and not cause.

Do you want a description, in Greek, of the parts of your body that are degenerating – or a diagnosis?

Because the diagnosis of ALS describes symptoms and not cause, drugs likewise treat symptoms and not cause. What if your car mechanic never fixed a problem, but only treated the symptoms? What if your car backfired and he put on a quieter muffler? What if the exhaust smoked and he installed a filter? Once you figured that out, would you go back to him?

As long as traditional medicine continues to treat symptoms rather than address cellular infection and nutritional deficiency, then the best the current system can offer is drugs to block or counteract the myriad of uncomfortable symptoms. The worst the current system can offer is unnecessary surgical procedures. It is not uncommon for people with autoimmune conditions to have multiple organs removed that were inflamed, infected and intractably painful. The inevitable knee-jerk reaction of chasing symptoms is: "If it hurts and we can't relieve the pain with drugs, then remove it."

To restore health means addressing the source of disease. *Disease* (dis-ease) means *lack of ease*. To restore health means rooting out the source of discomfort rather than symptomatically treating pain or supporting debilitation.

Allopathic medicine, which is practiced by MD's, aims to treat disease by the use of remedies which produce different effects from those which cause suffering by a disease ("allo" means "alternate" and "pathos" means "suffering"). This is why medical doctors often employ treatments but not cures. Elevated blood pressure is reduced with *anti*hypertensive medications, fever is reduced with a*nti*pyretic drugs and allergy related symptoms are suppressed with *anti*histamines.

In allopathy, the current treatment modalities for autoimmune conditions is based upon the theory that disease is due to an immune system gone haywire. Hence the goal of treatment is to block the immune system at various points in its communication and defense network.

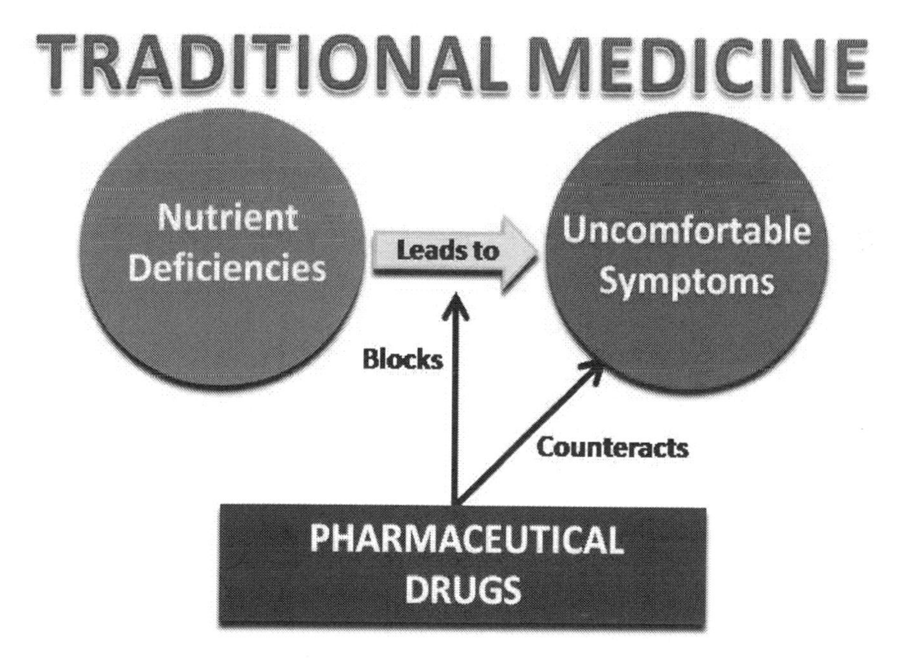

All of these medications simply *block* the body's reaction to insult and do not cure. Foundations supposedly dedicated to finding a cause for dreaded diseases have spent trillions of dollars in the last century as the list of degenerative and autoimmune diseases grows. Typically, 85% of the monies they raise are used for more fundraising.

Linus Pauling described a strange response from his employees when he discovered the vitamin C connection to cardiovascular disease. The hallways were quiet when he thought there would be shouts of joy. No one invested in looking for a cure really wants to work themselves out of a job by actually finding it!

While allopathic medicine certainly alleviates much suffering, relieving painful symptoms should not forever trump uncovering the root cause of disease. The "standard of care" should never be stubbornly implemented in the face of substantial data that provides plausible explanations for a multifactorial disease.

Let us, rather, put the axe to the root.

We are made of cells and organelles within cells that comprise organs and yet physicians largely specialize by organs. Chronic neurodegenerative inflammatory diseases like ALS that affect the function of the entire body must be investigated at the cellular level. It is at the level of the cell – and not organs – that can only account for common injury to multiple tissues and organs.

Traditional drug-based medicine, then, is the practice of treating disease by blocking or counteracting symptoms of disease with chemicals. Most pharmaceuticals used today either circumvent or short-cut normal biochemical processes. Like all other things in life such as accruing wealth or wisdom, there are no shortcuts that work in the long run.

Health restoration, on the other hand, is the practice of replacing deficiencies rather than suppressing symptoms.

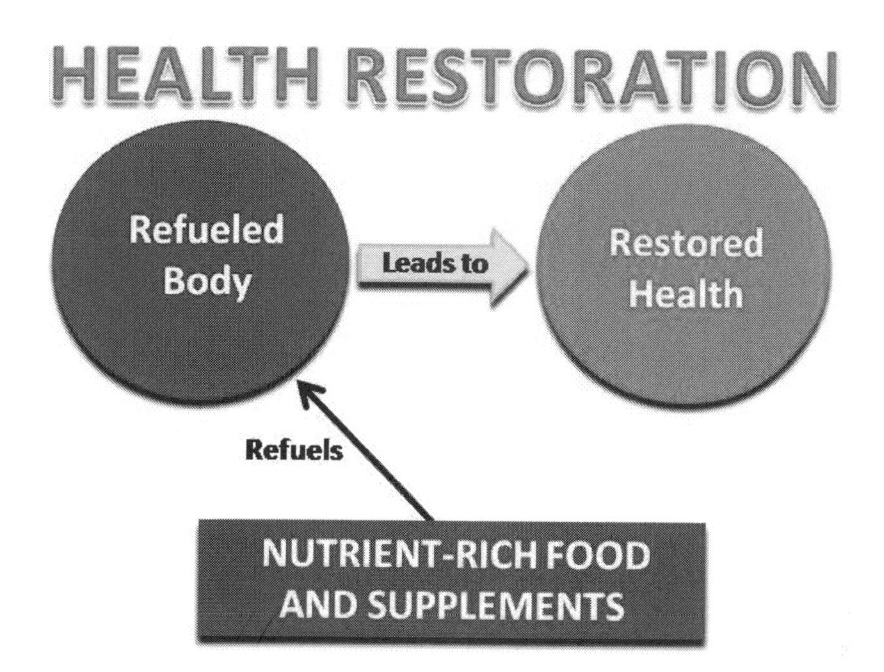

Rather than "treat" and "manage" disease, the focus in health restoration is on optimizing or returning to a normal state of cellular health. Scary names are not used, and the most useful test result is the answer to the question, "How do you feel?"

Bottom Line: Painful symptoms from deficiency states can be managed by blocking symptoms or surgically removing organs and tissues and thereby treating the disease, or can be managed by restoring cellular deficiencies and restoring health. ***This is the art and science of practicing cellular health.***

Chapter 3: Power of Hydrogen

"Health is worth more than learning."
-*Thomas Jefferson*

If you want to create a monumental amount of energy in a fraction of a second then split the hydrogen atom; this is called the hydrogen bomb.

Hydrogen – the tiniest atom on earth – is the source of energy for humans who are made of 50 to 70 percent water. Hydrogen, in turn, behaves predictably based on its water environment – *you*.

The *movement* of hydrogen through water depends upon a quality of water called the ***power of hydrogen***. This is important in conquering ALS because it is the movement of hydrogen in well oxygenated water that in large part makes for healthy cells. You are made up of billions upon billions of cells. Healthy, energized and well-oxygenated cells make for a healthy you.

The power of hydrogen, or pH, is a measurement of the amount of hydrogen in water using a logarithmic scale from 0 to 14. Water with a pH of 7 is *neutral*. Water with a pH less than 7 has increasing amounts of hydrogen and is *acidic*. Water with a pH greater than 7 has increasing amounts of oxygen and is *basic*.

The pH of blood (iron-colored "water") is normally maintained at an average 7.4 – just slightly basic.

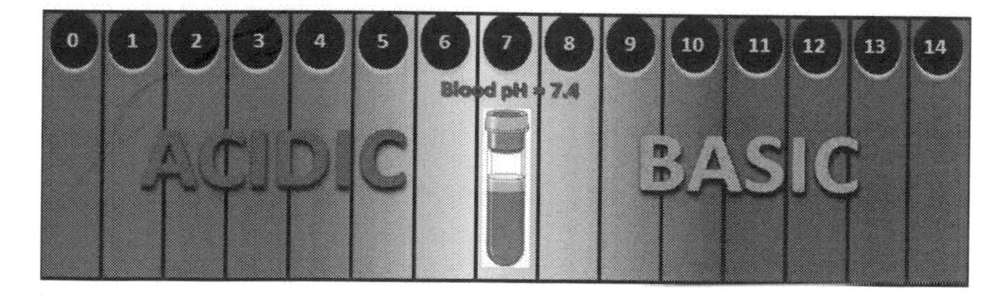

The slightly basic pH of human blood is VITAL to health. This is because a basic blood pH of 7.4 supports an oxygen-rich blood "bath" to cells, tissues and organs.

Water is H_2-O. Neutral water has two hydrogen atoms for every oxygen atom. Since acidic water contains more hydrogen than neutral water, acidic water has less oxygen than neutral water.

Correspondingly, basic water with a pH greater than 7 has more oxygen than neutral water – and cells require plenty of oxygen and nutrients to function normally.

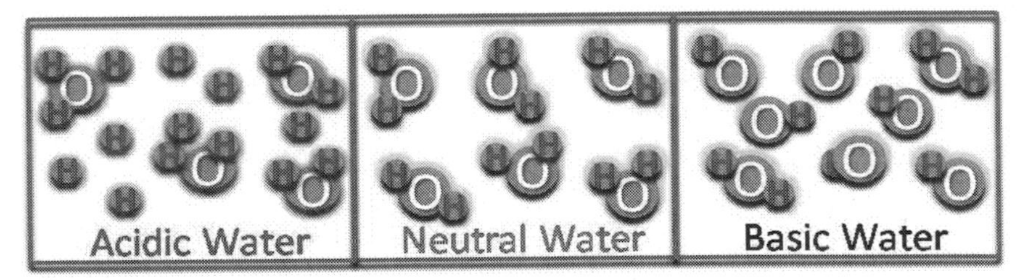

Why is this important? Human blood, cells, tissues and organs are 50-70% water, so the science that applies to keeping water at a well-oxygenated and life-promoting pH also applies to you.

Because there is more oxygen in basic water with a pH above 7, some athletes carefully monitor the pH of the fluids they drink to ensure their body water remains basic. With more oxygen, one has more "wind" and therefore enjoys optimized physical endurance. On the other hand, a person complaining of increasing breathlessness with simple activity such as walking up a flight of stairs may be suffering the many ills of increasingly acidic and oxygen-deficient body (tissue) water.

We are born basic and we die acidic – and so it is that we literally degenerate with age. Acid water in a cement swimming pool causes leaching of alkaline minerals such as calcium from the cement, which erodes the supporting structure.

Similarly, acid water in *you* causes leaching of calcium from bone and subsequent degeneration of the skeleton and teeth. The loss of minerals (calcium from bones, magnesium from muscle and sodium and potassium from cells) is at the root of many of the degenerative diseases associated with aging.

Interestingly, basic water with a pH above 7 is also *clean* water – and this is a vital life-enhancing quality of blood with a pH of 7.4. ***Only one simple test is required to keep a swimming pool clean: a pH test.*** Clean pool water is maintained at the same pH of normal human blood – a slightly basic pH of 7.4 which is just outside the acid range.

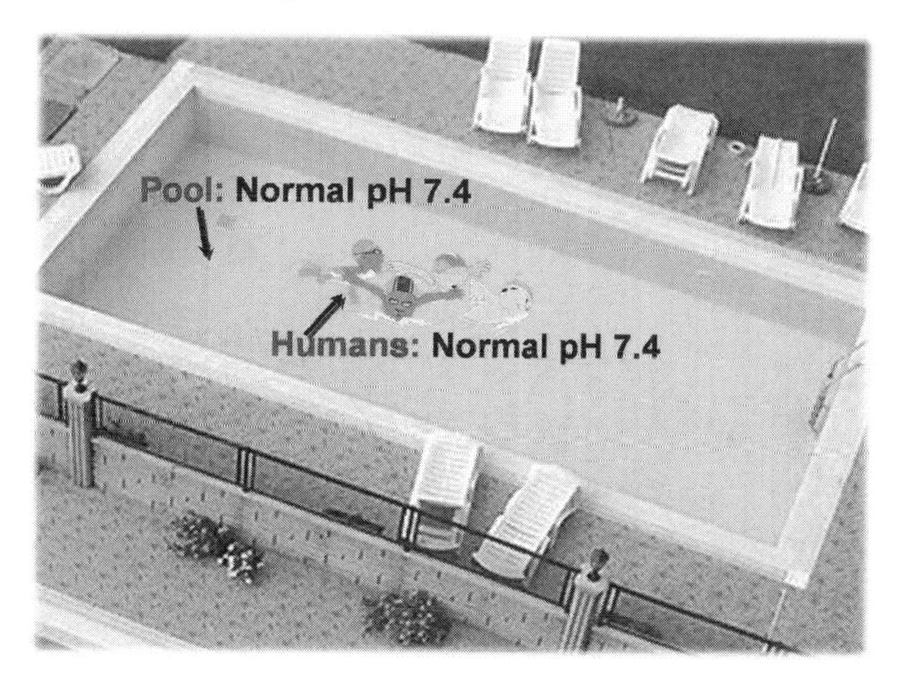

When the pH of water drops below 7, bacteria and fungi that love to grow in oxygen-deficient acidic water start to multiply and turn the water green. The microbes that thrive in acidic water and turn swimming pools into cesspools are primarily oxygen-hating *anaerobes* (*anaerobe* means *without oxygen*). The less oxygen or more acidic the water, the more anaerobic microbes can multiply.

A dirty malodorous pool of water reveals their growing presence!

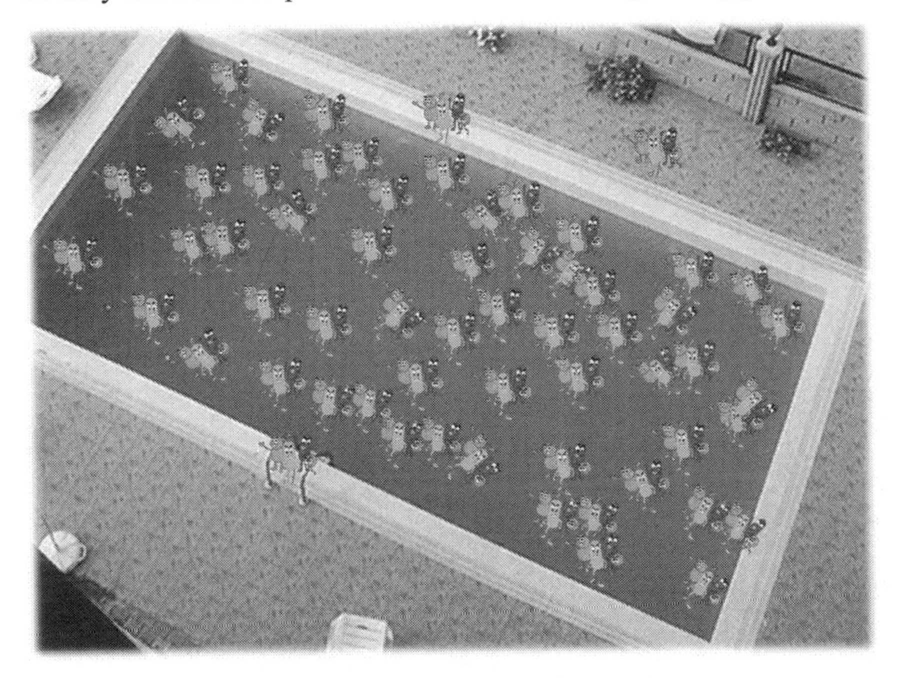

The solution? Sodium bicarbonate (baking soda), poured into a contaminated pool to raise the acidic pH back to a slightly basic 7.4, will kill the oxygen-hating, acid-loving and stinky anaerobes. No prescription antibiotics, designer drugs or expensive chemicals are required – just pH correction.

A slightly basic water pH of 7.4 is nature's antibiotic!

Your body, then, just like the careful owner of a swimming pool, regulates the pH of your blood to maintain a pH of 7.4. This is just above the acid range that acid-loving disease-causing bacteria and fungi love.

What do pH and anaerobic organisms have to do with anything regarding ALS? A whole lot! Acid-loving anaerobic organisms, which normally live in balance in a basic water pH, proliferate in an acidic pH because they hate oxygen. These anaerobes (such as Chlamydia, Mycoplasma and Ureaplasma) metabolize dietary carbohydrates – *but without needing oxygen.* The by-products of this are acids that in turn feed the acid-loving and oxygen-hating microbes, fueling an increasingly oxygen-deficient disease-promoting water inside of the swimming pool called *you.* The result is more and more anaerobes to rob you of your energy, wind (breath) and health that can only be attained and maintained in a basic water pH.

An acidic condition, though difficult to diagnose without taking a tissue biopsy to test the tissue bed pH, is repairable.

Now you know why autoimmunity and infection – especially recurrent bladder infections (in women) – go hand-in-hand. These anaerobic microbes are so tiny that they are undetected by most automated lab machines and are invisible under most microscopes – even electron microscopes. The diseases they cause are often left undiagnosed or sometimes attributed to an "autoimmune" condition.

Bottom Line: Basic water has more oxygen than acidic water. ***Slightly basic water with a pH of 7.4 is a nature's antibiotic to resist over-population of oxygen-hating, acid-generating, disease-causing and fat-promoting anaerobic microbes.***

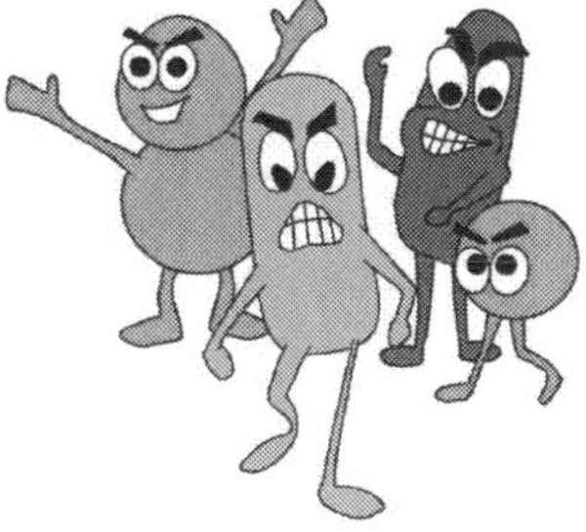

Chapter 4: Basics of Life

"It is health that is real wealth and not gold and silver."
-Mahatma Gandhi

It is interesting to note that humans have about the same ratio of water to tissue mass as the earth's water to land mass.

As it is on earth, water pH and life are interdependent. The pH of blood, which is mostly water, is closely regulated by the body to maintain a slightly basic (alkaline) pH of 7.4. This pH helps keep the blood free of pathogenic anaerobes and, more importantly, serves to *keep the heart and the brain working optimally*!

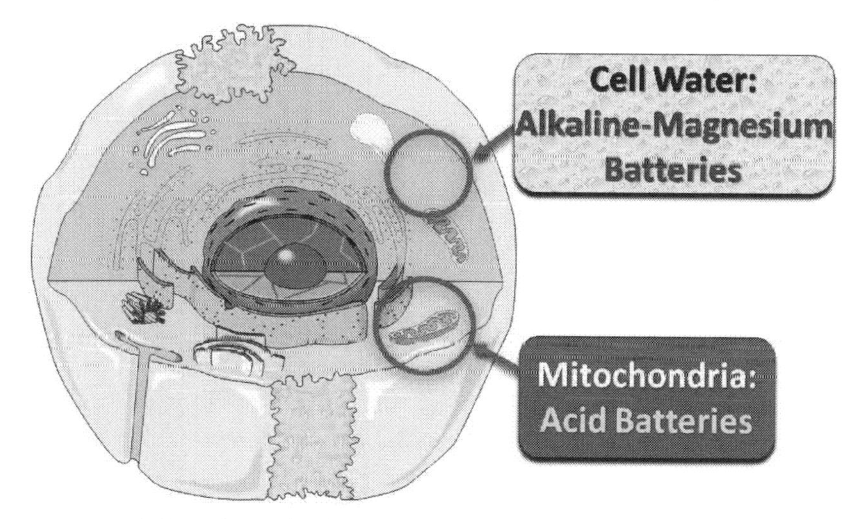

For normal function, the human heart and brain – the central processing units – are dependent upon a basic water pH, calcium and magnesium to promote hundreds of cellular reactions. The water matrix of cells is like an alkaline magnesium battery which supports life giving chemical reactions such as the contraction of heart cells and conduction of brain cells and nerves. On the other hand, the energy making mechanism of cells (inside peanut-shaped "mitochondria") is dependent upon an environment that is more like acid batteries housed within the basic cell water.

Despite the body tightly regulates a blood pH of 7.4 to support normal function of vital organs such as the heart and brain, physicians typically do not routinely check blood pH. On the other hand, "blood gas" tests are routinely ordered in medical emergencies such as heart attacks or comas induced by metabolic acidosis. Often, arterial blood pH will prove to be below normal.

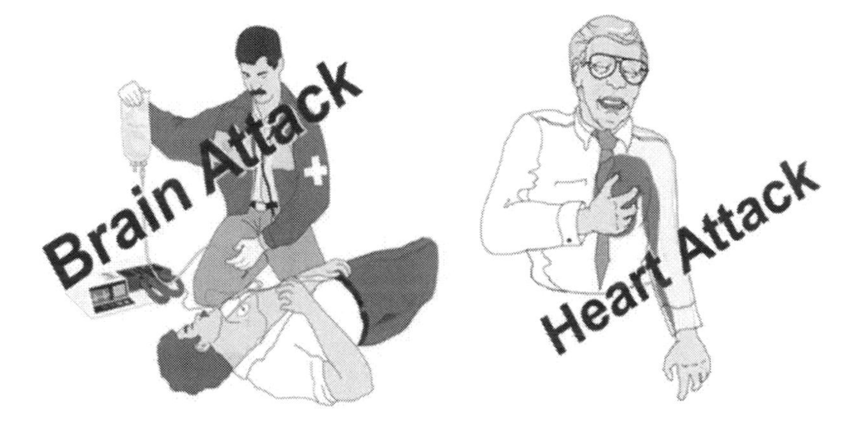

In animal experiments, a small but *rapid* drop in blood pH (such as from 7.4 to 7.2) results in rapid death by cardiac arrest. The blood pH of heart attack and diabetic coma victims, however, may be as low as 6.8 – ***revealing the body's ability to slowly compensate for an acidic environment over years.***

Alkaline mineral stores such as magnesium, calcium and potassium from muscles can also be mobilized to raise blood pH. A blood pH between 6.8 and 7.2 in a medical emergency such as a heart attack indicates that the body's pH regulatory mechanism has been overwhelmed by chronic depletion of alkaline mineral stores from muscle, bones and organs.

A basic blood pH of 7.4 is stabilized by positively charged alkaline minerals (sodium, potassium, magnesium and calcium) that neutralize negatively charged acids. Alkaline minerals, then, serve to keep a water pH above 7. Deep waters extracted from expansive mineral beds, for example, have been measured to have a basic pH above 9.

All waters, then, are not the same!

Since the human blood is carefully regulated at a basic pH of 7.4, the health risks of drinking trendy distilled water that is void of all minerals should be obvious. Distilled water has no minerals and is usually slightly acidic. It is not the slightly acidic pH of distilled water, however, that is a health risk; *it is absence of minerals*.

Water drunk on an empty stomach is absorbed directly into arterial blood that delivers nutrients and oxygens to the organs and tissues of the body. When distilled water is absorbed into the blood, the body is hard-wired to mobilize alkaline minerals from various tissue beds and organ stores to protect the life supporting blood pH of 7.4. This is essential to protect the heart, which requires a mineral-rich basic blood-bath. ***Tissues and organs are robbed of mineral stores to protect the blood pH so as to preserve heart and brain function.***

Never drink distilled water. Protect the mineral stores in your muscles and bones – there's no need to degenerate sooner than later!

What about soda? 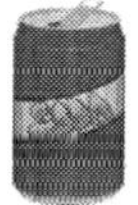

The incalculable health risk of drinking soda as a thirst quencher is found in its acidity. The measurement of pH is a logarithmic scale in which every decreasing unit of pH has 10 times more hydrogen. Water with a pH of 7 is neutral. Water with a pH of 6 has 10 times more hydrogen than water with a pH of 7. Water with a pH of 5 has 100 times more hydrogen than a pH of 7. Water with a pH of 4 has 1,000 times more hydrogen than water with a pH of 7 and so on. More hydrogen means more acid.

The pH of healthy human blood is 7.4. The pH of soda is 3.4. The difference between 7.4 and 3.4 is 4.0 which, on a logarithmic scale, is ten times ten times ten times ten (that's four tens or 10^4).

In other words, soda is 10,000 times more acidic than blood!

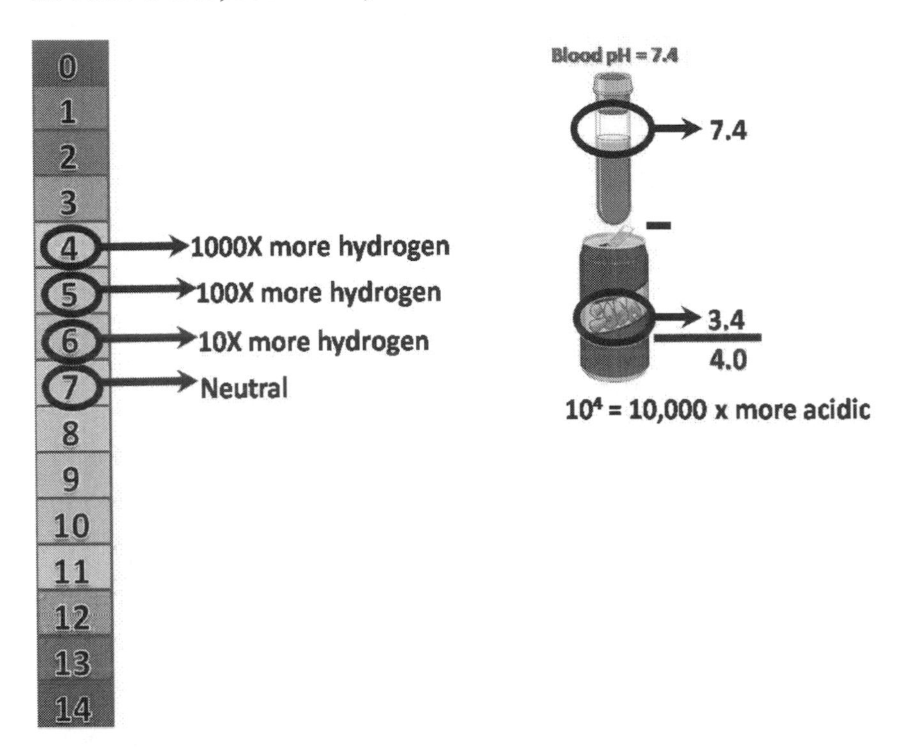

Like soda, the pH of grapefruit and orange juice is also 3.4. The acidity of these natural juices, however, is from *citric acid* which is a metabolic super-fuel that promotes a basic blood pH by fueling the citric acid cycle and promoting complete oxidation of carbohydrates (much more on this later). ***The acidity of most sodas, on the other hand, is from phosphoric acid, which is a strong oxidizer, destroys cells membranes, and robs the body of calcium and oxygen.*** This promotes an acid environment for pathogenic microbes to enjoy and further degenerate cells.

Bottom Line: Human blood is carefully regulated at a basic pH of 7.4. A chronically-acidic blood pH can eventually cause cardiac arrest and make a cesspool for acid-loving microbes.

Chapter 5: Soda Pop and Popping Joints

"Every human being is the author of his own health or disease."
-Buddha

Soda is 10,000 times more acidic than blood. No wonder it worked so well as a child to clean up collectible pennies! The question that begs to be asked is: ***Why would we drink an oxidizing metal cleaner, give it to our children and not think it could harm us?***

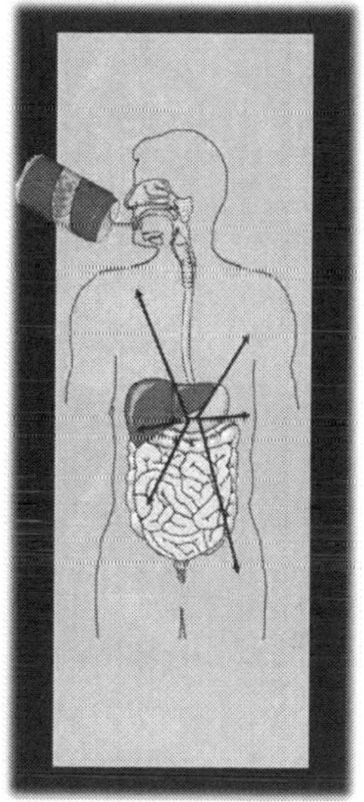

The acidity of soda is often overlooked as a main contributor to autoimmune and degenerative diseases. Many people reason that because the pH of stomach acid is lower than the pH of soda, soda must be safe to drink! What is missed is that there is no release of stomach acid when soda is drunk on an empty stomach. Instead, it is directly absorbed into the blood via the arteries that line the stomach and first part of the small intestine. This takes only minutes.

Included with all that processed sugar or artificial sweetener (choose your poison) is a whopping bolus of *phosphoric acid* that directly enters the bloodstream and instantly reacts with dissolved calcium in the blood. This is a predictable and reproducible chemical reaction because phosphoric acid has a strong negative charge that is neutralized by the strong positive charge of ionized calcium in blood (like lightening to ground, nature always seeks electrical neutrality). The product of this reaction is calcium phosphate that is filtered through the kidneys and discharged in the urine.

If excessive calcium phosphate is formed so that it can no longer remain dissolved in blood, calcium phosphate kidney stones can precipitate.

The physiological response to a drop in dissolved calcium in the blood is a release of parathyroid hormone from the parathyroid glands. Parathyroid hormone stimulates removal of calcium from bone to replace the calcium that's been lost from the blood. With insufficient calcium in the diet to compensate for the loss of calcium to the greedy bonds of phosphoric acid, bone loss is the predictable result.

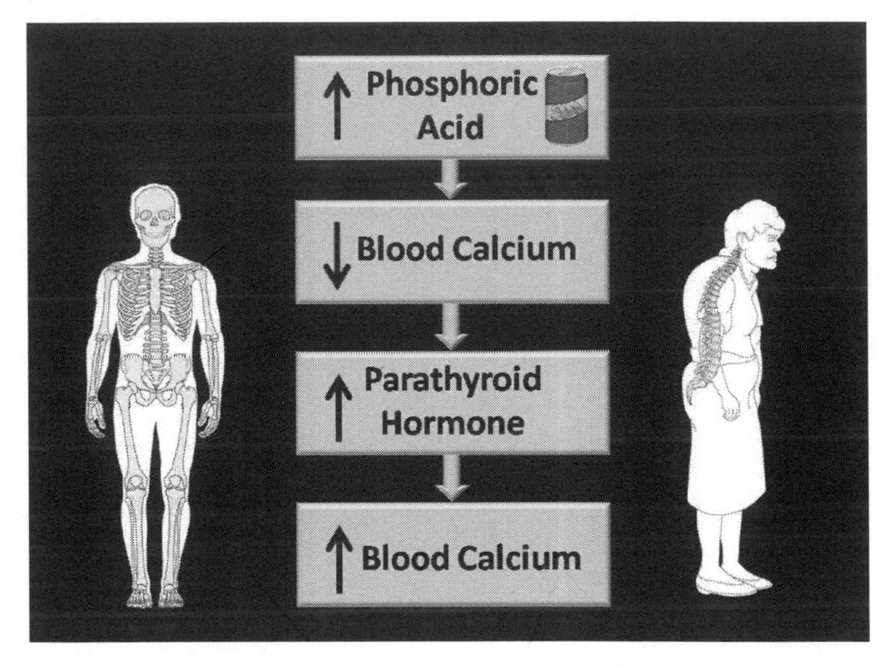

There's no way to predict the long-term effects of phosphoric acid soft drinks, since the body quickly neutralizes this extra acid with dissolved calcium in the blood and then mobilizes calcium carbonate (from bone) to neutralize any remaining extra acid. In other words, the pH of blood quickly returns to normal to protect the heart and brain...but at what expense *?N*o one knows or cared to consider and measure when soda was approved for human consumption.

Theoretically, one too many glasses of soda drunk on an empty stomach could stop the heart from a rapid drop in pH. There are no reported deaths attributed to a soda drinking competition. Nevertheless, most every medical doctor has performed this simple pH experiment by arresting the heart of lab dogs with acid directly injected into arterial blood.

Drinking soda with food, on the other hand, is physiologically safer because the food mixes with hydrochloric acid in the stomach (which is 100 times stronger than the acid in soda) and then the mixture moves into the first part of the small intestines ***where the alkaline-rich enzymes of the pancreas neutralize everything – including the soda.***

Nevertheless, despite soda drunk with food will minimize the pH-drop in blood that happens when soda is drunk on an empty stomach, the phosphoric acid will still bind calcium in food – and if not in the food, in blood! Mixing milk with soda minimizes this because the calcium in the milk, rather than the calcium in blood, will instantly react with the phosphoric acid.

Calcium is a remarkable alkalinizing mineral that reacts with water in the blood and causes hydrogen molecules to off-gas. ***The result is water with a more basic pH that buffers (protects) the blood from a drop in pH with ingestion of acids.***

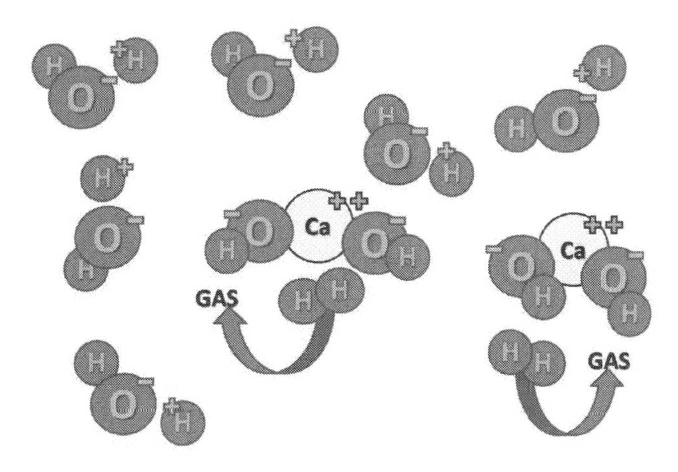

Drinking soda with phosphoric acid depletes the pH-protective quality of calcium – by eliminating it! Phosphoric acid reacts with calcium and removes it from the blood, thus depleting the body's most valuable mineral resource for regulating a life sustaining oxygen-rich basic blood pH of 7.4.

Do you wonder at what point the body stops removing calcium from bone so as to keep a skeleton from turning to mush? Surely the exquisite human endocrine system would at some point spare the bone and instead compromise calcium-rich tissue beds like muscle. Magnesium stores in bone and muscle are also, in time, depleted. This does happen. People routinely show up in emergency rooms with acidic blood, arrested hearts, degenerating skeletons and stiff and sore muscles.

Calcium is not the only mineral with which phosphoric acid instantly reacts; it also reacts with magnesium to form magnesium phosphate. Magnesium is found in the blood, bone *and in muscle*. Magnesium stores in the muscle and bone replace depleted blood magnesium that reacts with and neutralizes phosphoric acid.

Muscles and nerves require calcium and magnesium to function.

So, with soda pop on most every table in first-world countries, and popping joints, degenerative disease, fibromyalgia, kidney stones and all kinds of strange "autoimmune" conditions like ALS skyrocketing through the roof who knows how much disease that soda with 10,000 times more acidity than human blood has caused. Remarkably, over 23 million Americans have been diagnosed with some kind of degenerative and/or inflammatory disease of unknown origin.

Bottom Line: Phosphoric acid sodas deplete blood calcium and magnesium which normally alkalinize blood to maintain a healthy life supporting basic pH of 7.4. Basic blood has more oxygen to support metabolism. ***Do not drink soft drinks – ever.***

Chapter 6: Contaminated Pools

"To wish to be well is part of becoming well."
-Seneca

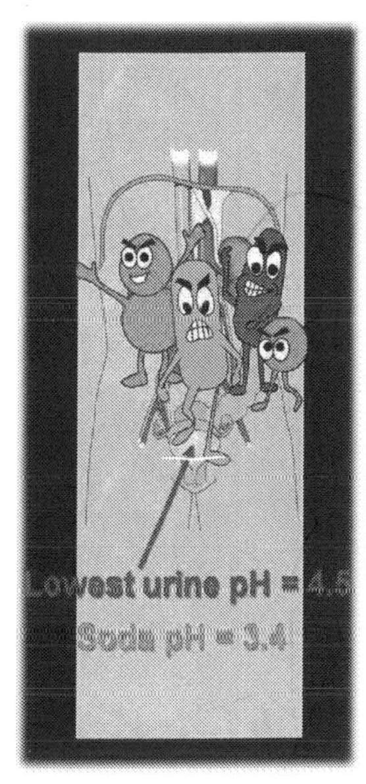

If the risks of kidney stones and bone loss are insufficient reason to reclassify soft drinks as metal and porcelain cleaners, at least the acidity of soda should have raised a few red flags from the scientific community over a century ago.

Human kidneys can only acidify urine to a pH of 4.5 and the pH of soda is 3.4 which is still ten times more acidic than the lowest urine pH! These connections were never made because the bone degenerating and muscle debilitating effects of drinking phosphoric acid surface so slowly that the cause and effect link is missed.

Acidic fresh-squeezed and unpasteurized fruit juices with a corresponding pH of soda are loaded with alkaline minerals and vitamins so that, when metabolized, they promote a basic rather than acidic pH. ***This is not the case with soda.*** If you ingest more acidic substances than your body can remove, the acid has nowhere to go but into organs and tissues – and acidic waters not only make muscles hurt but they are a natural environment for tiny anaerobic microbes to multiply and have a hay-day inside the water called *you*, going largely undetected by the most advanced medical laboratory tests.

Remember all those acid-loving anaerobic organisms that proliferate in an acidic swimming pool? In the urinary tract, these stealth oxygen-hating pathogens (such as Ureaplasma) are undetected by routine urinalysis machines. Because they are so small – only about 1/100th the size of a cell – they literally slip through microscopes and urine tests, left unseen and unmeasured. Medical providers more often than not, do not consider specialty tests for these microbes, because they are normally found in humans and all living things including animals, plants and insects. In acidic waters, however, they can be lethal to cells.

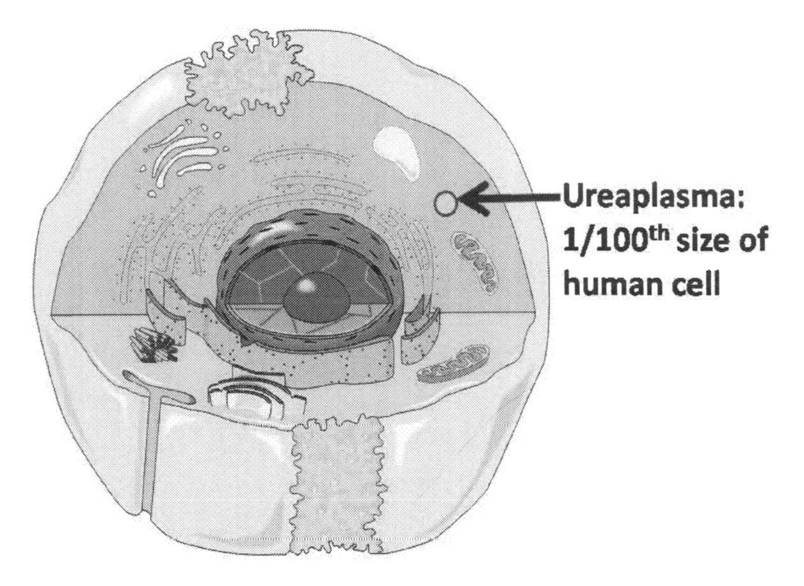

What is *not* normal, however, is for normal flora to become opportunistic pathogens by over-proliferating in an abnormally acidic environment. But, just because microbes cannot be seen or measured in someone complaining of chronic bladder irritation, chronic prostate inflammation or chronic muscle weakness – *does not mean they are not there*!

In acidic water, normally-balanced microbes can become disease-causing pathogens. *Anaerobic* microorganisms can only make energy *anaerobically* – which means "without oxygen". The end products of this are more acids which, in turn, further support the acid-loving parasites.

With a rise in autoimmune disease has also been an increase in "contaminants" of anaerobic microbes (Mycoplasma, Ureaplasma and Chlamydia) growing in clinical samples of human blood, urine and tissues. Despite common thinking, these pesky little bugs growing amuck in lab samples are NOT contaminants from the air or lab technicians. ***Many are "autoimmune" disease causing pathogens resident in the lab samples!***

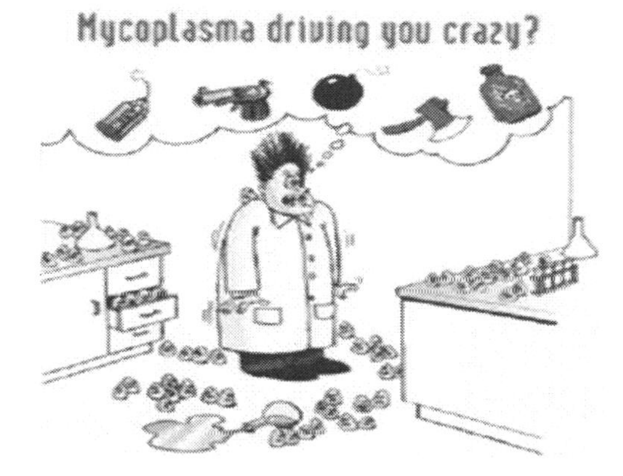

Mycoplasma and Ureaplasma cannot be seen by regular microscopes. Live blood analysis, on the other hand, such as dark-field microscopy (which is typically not used in western medicine), brings these life-forms into view. They are part of normal blood – ***and most doctors don't even know they are normally present in blood, tissues and organs!***

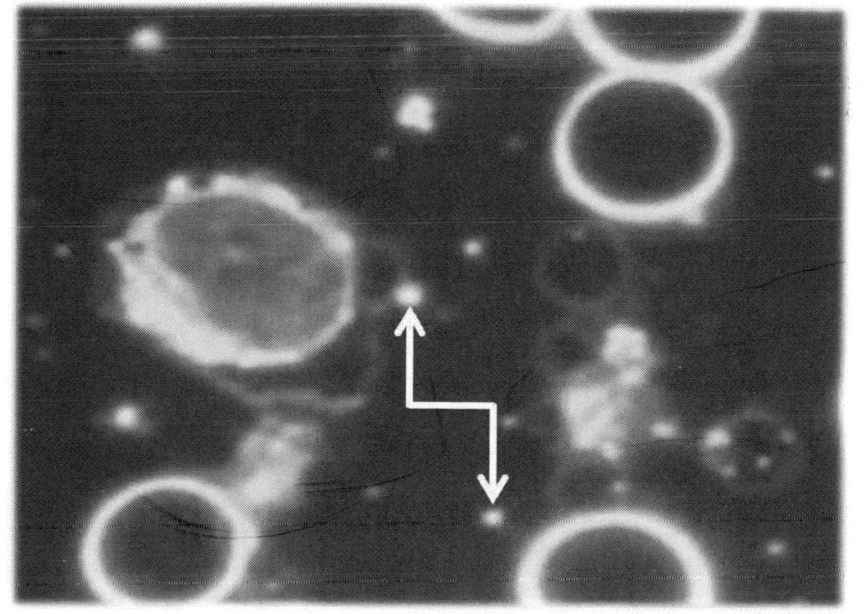

While little is known about these tiny single-celled microbes, they seem connected to the immune system and are very active around white blood cells. An educational video of this "activity" is posted at YouTube.com ("Earth's Tiniest Living Organisms"). When we die and no longer breathe oxygen, they yet live without oxygen – turning a body to dust even though sealed in a casket.

Death, the final degenerative disease of man, represents the ultimate acidic condition of our bodies – and these microbes thrive in acid water. ***What do these microbes do to us when our body water becomes acidic and mimics the condition of death?***

Electron microscopy points to the answer – that these microbes simply do their job and clean up the garbage of degenerating cells and tissues. Under a regular microscope this cell would appear abnormal, but likely dismissed without concern and given the description "poikilocytosis" which means "lots of pokey things" on the cell surface. But the scanning electron microscope reveals hundreds of anaerobic Mycoplasma coating the white blood cell!

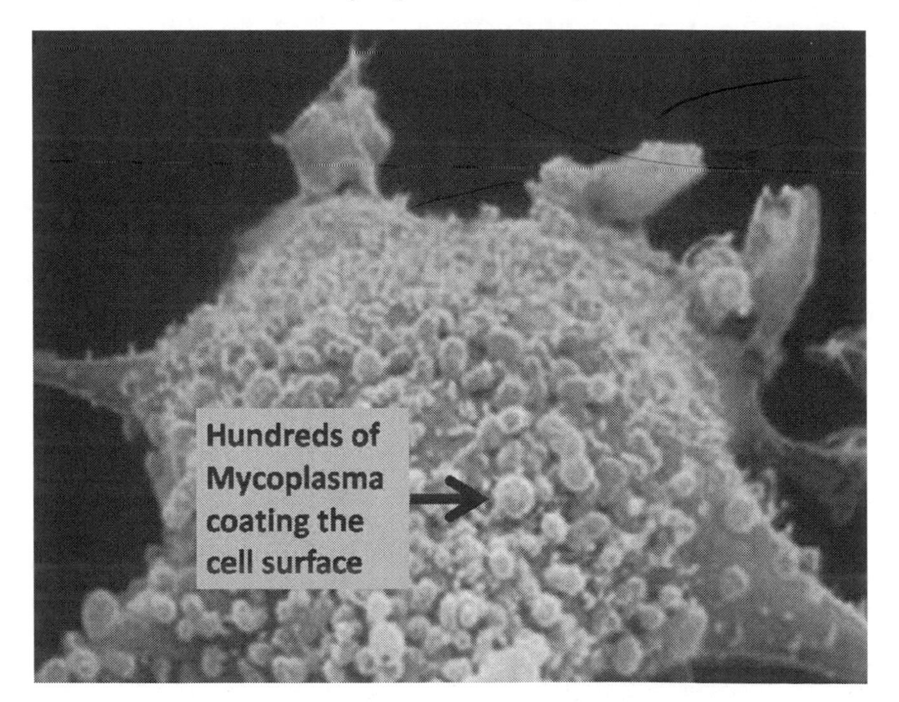

Case reports and classical studies have implicated these microbes in almost every "autoimmune" disease known to man (references 1-20) – including ALS.

"Autoimmune" means that the white blood cells of the immune system attack and destroy cells: muscle cells, thyroid cells, joint synovium, etc. In ALS, the immune system appears to be destroying the outer myelin sheath of nerves – causing "multiple scars" ("Amyotrophic Lateral Sclerosis") in the central nervous system.

This is deceiving to doctors and scientists alike. The appearance of white blood cells at the site of the problem is a symptom and not cause of the problem.

What is notable about earth's tiniest organisms – Mycoplasma, Ureaplasma and Chlamydia – is that unlike most bacteria, they lack a rigid cell wall. ***They are a unique class of single-celled microbes called Cell Wall Deficient (CWD) bacteria***.

I will use the term "CWD bacteria" throughout this book to describe these unusual tiny microbes with cholesterol-rich jellyfish-like plasma cell membranes that constantly change shape. (Again, most bacteria, fungi and viruses have rigid cell walls!) Also, most CWD bacteria lack the genes to make essential molecules like cholesterol to keep their mobile membranes intact. ***Inevitably, they are most commonly found invading cholesterol-rich cells and tissues: muscle cells, thyroid cells, joints and nerves.***

CWD bacteria are able to invade the INSIDE of cells!

Is the immune system really attacking inappropriately as doctors commonly think – or is the immune system simply doing its job by trying to attack the invaders and clean up "infected" tissue? In my book, the immune system is exquisitely engineered. You won't catch me prescribing immune-suppressing cytotoxic drugs to prevent someone's immune system from trying to do its job!

If CWD bacteria are like mosquitoes contaminating stagnant water, then the question begs to be asked: "***Do mosquitoes contaminate water, or do mosquitoes show up because the water is contaminated?***"

If the latter is correct, then correcting the acidic water will bring the body back into balance. Like cleaning dirty water in a pool, pH correction is nature's most potent antibiotic.

Bottom Line: Excess dietary acid stored up in tissues sets up an opportunistic environment for anaerobic microorganisms to over-proliferate and invade host cells. These unseen and undetected microbes metabolize food into acids, making increasingly acidic body waters in which they thrive.

Chapter 7: The ALS Infection Connection

"Facts do not cease to exist, just because they are ignored."
-Aldous Huxley

Autoimmune diseases, like cardiovascular diseases, have been on the rise since the turn of the 20th century when chlorination of public water supplies and soft drinks became popular. Notably, chlorine and phosphoric acid are acidic oxidizers that destroy cell membranes and compromise the body's normal basic pH. Marine lifeforms quickly die in a chlorinated pool.

If you poured a bunch of soft drinks into a swimming pool it wouldn't take long for it to look slimy-green – so why pour it into you? The filth of a dirty swimming pool represents a factory of acid-loving microbes that will, in time, degenerate a pool.

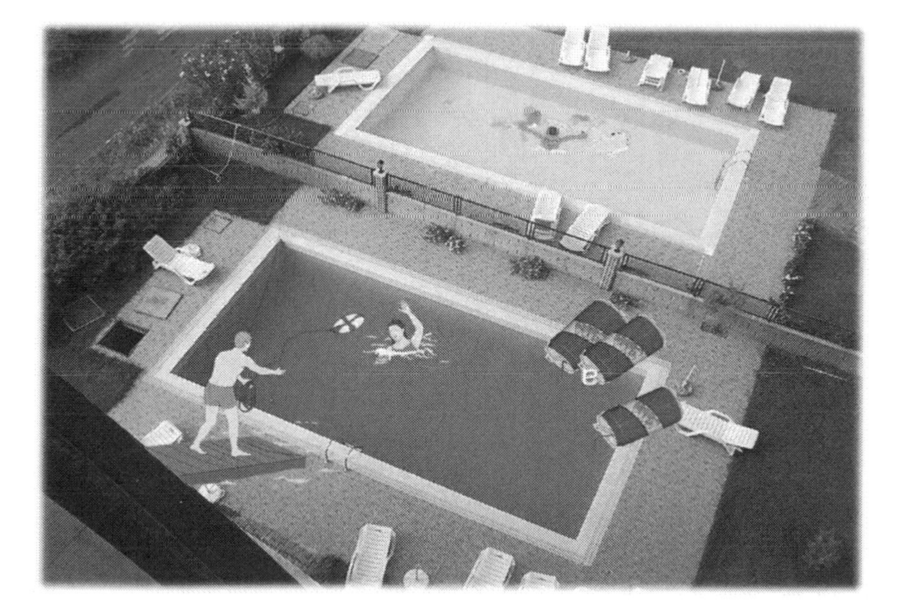

Unlike testing pool water with a simple pH paper strip, there is no accurate way to test the pH of human tissues. We can test blood, but it is almost always a predictable 7.4 until the mineral reserves of muscle and bone have been depleted. Even so, the tiny microbes that contaminate pools can also infect us. Just because doctors don't know about them, or don't test for them (or do test for them but think they are "lab contaminants"), doesn't mean they they can't and don't thrive in us under the right conditions. Not unlike phosphoric acid sodas, nutrient deficient foods also contaminate our "swimming pools" with dietary acids and further feed the bugs (more on that in Part Two).

These tiny organisms frequently infect the urinary tract and are a recurrent problem in females with ALS. Again, they are usually undetected by most lab equipment but frequent urinary infections are another tell-tale sign of a long-standing "stealth" infection by CWD anaerobic bacteria.

CWD bacteria can cross the blood-brain barrier and get into the spinal cord. They are so tiny that hundreds to thousands of them can grow INSIDE human cells. Human cells are a host for them because they can not make life-essential molecules like cholesterol. They then steal them from the host cells; they are intracellular parasites. Cholesterol is a vital part of the nervous system – and CWD bacteria need lots of cholesterol.
An activated immune system in the face of an undetected infection and damaged cells is not an abnormal "autoimmune" response!!! Elevated white blood cells, rather, are a sign that the immune system is simply trying to do its job.

While suppressing the immune system with drugs can slow down the destructive effects of white blood cells that are attacking nerve cells, only symptoms are blocked. The immune system has a real enemy to destroy – and immunosuppressive drugs hamstring the immune system! Over time, there is also risk of blindness from cataracts, liver disease and a whole host of other dangerous effects from these drugs. ***The problem of CWD bacteria hiding inside cells – and the toxins they make and release when host cells die – is not addressed.***

In ALS, there is supporting evidence for a very real but hidden infection within the fluid and cells of the nervous system. These include Chlamydia pneumoniae and various species of pathogenic Mycoplasma:

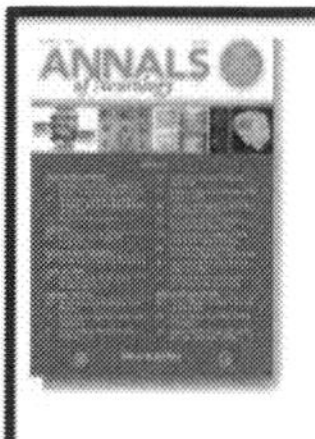

Presence of Chlamydia pneuomoniae DNA in the Cerebral Spinal Fluid is a Common Phenomenon in a Variety of Neurological Diseases and not Restricted to MS

Annals of Neurology, 2001: 49 (5): 585-589

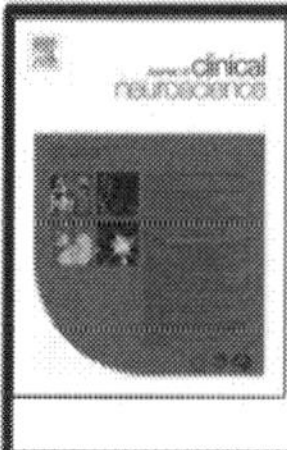

High Frequency of Systemic Mycoplasmal Infections in Gulf War Veterans and Civilians with Amyotrophic Lateral Sclerosis

Journal of Clinical Neuroscience, 2002: 9: 525-29.

Infectious Disease Newsletter 2007

Systemic Intracellular Bacterial Infections (*Mycoplasma, Chlamydia, Borrelia* species) in Neurodegenerative (MS, ALS) and Behavioral Disorders (ASD)

Garth L. Nicolson

The Institute for Molecular Medicine
16371 Gothard Street H
Huntington Beach, California 92647

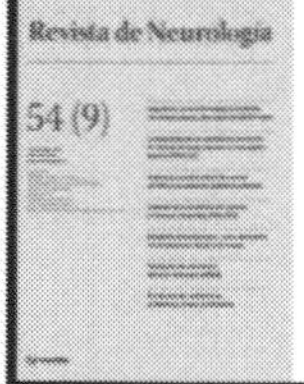

Determination of Systemic Infections due to Mycoplasma in Patients with Clinically Defined Amyotrophic Lateral Sclerosis

Rev Neurol., 2005: 41 (5): 262-67

Unlike bacteria with cell walls, CWD bacteria change into different forms during their life cycle. For example, in its early fungal-like spore or "elementary bodies" stage, Chlamydia pneumoniae can spread throughout the body via the bloodstream. Once a spore penetrates a cell it morphs into its more bacteria-like "reticulate bodies" stage. Here, the organism saps the cell's energy to reproduce more microbes that then hibernate (cryptic stage). In time, Chlamydia pneumoniae toxins destroy the host cell; this releases elementary bodies and toxins into the bloodstream. The released spores then infect more cells.

Once diagnosed, CWD bacteria may be treated with a combined antibiotic/antifungal regimen (doxycycline, ciprofloxicin, diflucan and/or tamoxifen). This can cause great discomfort for the patient because they produce toxins that are released when killed. These toxins, which kill host cells and gliocytes (which make myelin to protect nerves) by apoptosis, can exacerbate inflammation and make a person feel much worse before better.

The alternative, immunosuppression, is no sensible alternative. Antibiotics, antifungals and immune-suppressing drugs also do not completely address root cause. Again, mosquitoes do not pollute water; rather, they infest water that's already foul. Cleaning up stagnant water is a safer and more lasting alternative to insecticides to permanently oust "mosquitoes".

Build it (bad food and oxidizing drink), they will come. Remove it (bad food and drink), they will leave and/or not come. In other words, ***"Let food be your medicine and medicine be your food".***

Statin drugs for lowering cholesterol are also a BAD idea for anyone diagnosed with ALS. Statins are associated with drug-induced ALS. Symptoms of myelin loss in ALS is further compounded by blocking cholesterol with a statin drug because myelin is made from cholesterol.

As you will see in chapters 10 and 11, statins are similar to other fungal/CWD bacteria toxins that cause direct damage and death to nerve cells leaving multiple "scars" (sclerosis). *Do not take them!*

The most disruptive substances to restoring cells back to normal health are:

1. Statin drugs (and other immune suppressing drugs)
2. Soft drinks and chlorinated water
3. Smoke (tobacco, etc.)
4. Sham foods (processed carbohydrates)

Do not take these if health restoration is your goal.

Bottom Line: Tiny CWD bacteria, the smallest organisms in the world and normally found in blood, can turn into disease-causing parasitic pathogens in a low-oxygen (anaerobic) acidic water environment. Just because doctors do not know about them, or do not test for them, ***does not mean they are not there!***

Chapter 8: Serial Killers

"Healing is a matter of time,
but it is also a matter of opportunity."
-Hippocrates

Imagine waking up to breakfast in bed; seated on your lap is a tray of delights like hot apple cider with cinnamon, scrumptious scrambled eggs, fresh sliced tomatoes, tender baby carrot sticks and a bouquet of red roses. Those sights, smells and savory flavors are samples of nature's marvelous *isoprenoids*.

Isoprenoids are the largest and most diverse class of over 25,000 molecules made by plants and animals. Because of isoprenoids, we can wake up and smell the roses, enjoy the spice of life (cinnamon), relish color (orange carrots and red tomatoes) and see it all clearly (vitamin A). Isoprenoids also include powerful antioxidants (vitamin E) with anti-cancer and heart-protective properties. One of the most villainized isoprenoids is cholesterol.

Vital to supporting life, isoprenoids support cell functions like metabolism, replication and membrane stability. If isoprenoid synthesis in cells is blocked, or if isoprenoids inside cells are destroyed, cells die.

Nearly all plants, animals and microbes make isoprenoids, but CWD bacteria like Chlamydia pneumoniae have lost the ability to make them. ***To survive, they invade cells and cause disease by stealing isoprenoids like cholesterol from the host.*** The malaria parasite likewise invades and scavenges cholesterol from red blood cells (reference 21). While foods rich in isoprenoids (the breakfast in bed example) may feed CWD bacteria, they also help replace the stolen "goods".

Isoprenoids are five-carbon fatty molecules. The myelin coat of nerves is rich with isoprenoids like cholesterol and dolichol.

Chlamydia pneumoniae can not survive without fatty isoprenoids like cholesterol and dolichol to grow its flexible membrane and to replicate. The nervous system is a rich source of their vital food.

Chlamydia pneumoniae are isoprenoid sapping parasites! Without isoprenoids, human cells also die. Small wonder the immune system *seemingly* attacks normal cells – because they aren't normal! Those cells are, rather infected, isoprenoid depleted, dying and dead cells. ***The immune system has not gone awry; it is doing exactly what it is exquisitely designed to do: destroy foreign invaders and clean up dead and dying tissue.***

Chlamydia pneumoniae may start as a respiratory tract infection like bronchitis and then travel to other parts of the body. Its spore-like fungal form is so tiny, it can pass through the blood-brain barrier that normally prevents microbes from infiltrating the the brain and spinal cord. The cells they invade are rich in the fatty isoprenoids they need to survive: nerve tissue, muscle cells, brain cells, the lining of blood vessels and the cholesterol-rich white blood cells (macrophages) of the immune system.

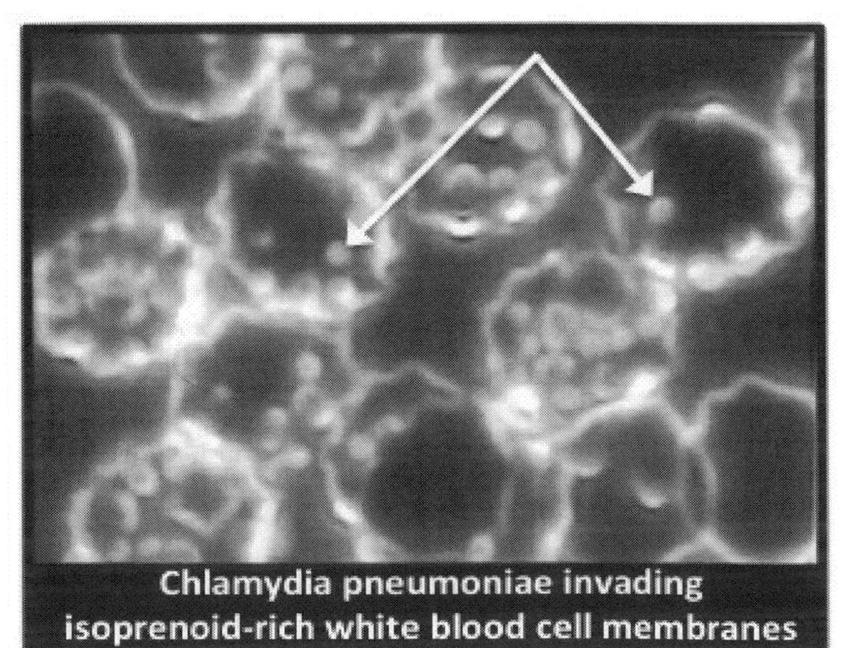
Chlamydia pneumoniae invading isoprenoid-rich white blood cell membranes

Chlamydia pneumoniae infection has been more frequently associated with MS than ALS. Mycoplasma infections are more frequently identified in ALS patients than MS patients. Oftentimes, multiple CWD bacteria are found by investigators who study the neurodegenerative "autoimmune" diseases. Because ALS, MS and other nerve degenerating syndromes represent a spectrum of disease with no clear-cut lines, making a definitive diagnosis can be difficult.

Physicians rarely test for CWD bacteria; most doctors have not even heard about them. Even if your doctor takes blood, urine and CSF samples, under a microscope no microbes will be seen. In lab cultures, these CWD bacteria might grow, but lab technicians have been trained to think they are environmental "contaminants". When found, antibiotics are added to the cultures in which they grow, and, like wiping away fingerprints from the scene of a crime, the incriminating evidence is willfully (albeit ignorantly) destroyed.

Doctors have been trained to "treat" autoimmune diseases based upon theory, not fact. The most widely accepted theory is that autoimmunity is triggered by allergens or viruses with similar proteins to normal tissue. The immune system then "confuses" normal tissue for a virus or other foreign invader and attacks normal cells. In this light, "auto-immune" means "self-immunity". In other words, the immune system doesn't know what it is doing and inadvertently attacks the host. In the case of ALS, the cells that are attacked are primary peripheral motor nerves (nerves that originate in the spinal cord and innervate muscles).

Immune suppressing drugs generally do not help with ALS, and current treatments which only help alleviate symptoms extend life by only months.

Current paradigms do not work. This is indisputable; if you have ALS then I am preaching to the choir. The current theory(s) supporting the current standards of care are *wrong*. Improved results are never going to found by doing the same old thing. Yet medicine in its current configuration is so badly broken with drug company interests driving medical protocols that it is probably irreparable; change is unlikely to come – if at all – as long as medicine remains a for-profit commodity. Inevitably, patients with so-called "autoimmune" illnesses are bounced from one doctor to the next, tossed expensive drugs that only alleviate some symptoms and/or subjected to untold needless surgeries.

It is spiraling out of control; this is part of the "healthcare crisis".

Occasionally, a reasonable physician will test an ALS patient for a CWD bacterial infection and, if a positive test is obtained, treat ALS with a combination of antibiotics and antifungals that will target the microbe in its various life cycle stages. Sadly, most physicians are simply too afraid to test or treat an illness outside mainstream practices. They fear losing licensure by not following the current "standard of care". There is safety in numbers, even if the numbers are all wrong. Who's running the show, anyway? (Follow the money.)

Furthermore, autoimmune disease symptoms are not clear cut, and doctors often disagree on a diagnosis. While MS and ALS both reveal "scars" on the myelin sheath surrounding nerves, some believe that only MS is an inflammatory and autoimmune process while ALS is not; others disagree and provide evidence to support that the immune system (white blood cells) are activated in ALS. Some say that MS involves primarily the CNS while ALS involves primarily the peripheral nerves. Sometimes ALS is called muscular atrophy which is confused for muscular dystrophy. And on and on the controversy goes, all in an attempt to clearly categorize nerve and muscle related degenerative diseases into their neat and tidy respective boxes.

The lack of agreement among investigators is evidence that the neuromuscular diseases are not as discrete as imagined by MD's, but are a spectrum of disease. Physicians are literally ridiculed from a path of discovery. It is not just what they learn – it is how they are taught; doctors are expected to have distinct diagnoses and protocols at the tip of their tongue while training, or they are passed over. Evidence-based medicine, based largely on evidence engineered by drug companies, has become fear-driven medicine.

Medical training is the most stifling educational process on earth. MD's are not taught to venture beyond the current drug-driven, disease-naming, fear-mongering and sickness-selling standards. ***Worse, they know little to nothing about CWD bacteria and the toxins they make.*** Since these microbes hide inside cells and invade multiple cell types, they cause a vast array of symptoms throughout the whole body.

This makes a correct diagnosis virtually impossible for a physician to make. But just because doctors remain largely uninformed of the matter does not mean pathogenic CWD bacterial toxins are not killing cells.

Another CWD bacteria linked with ALS is an isoprenoid thief like Chlamydia pneumoniae called *Mycoplasma pneumoniae*. Like Chlamydia, it has various life cycle stages and causes an "atypical" pneumoniae. A fraction the size of a human cell and also without a cell wall, it can infect most any type of cell. It most commonly afflicts the central nervous system:

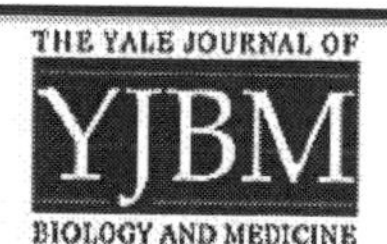

The Yale Journal of Biology and Medicine

1983: 56 (5-6): 475-9. Fernald G.W.

"Numerous case reports and retrospective studies suggest an association between Mycoplasma pneumoniae respiratory infection and extrapulmonary complications, the most common of which involve the central nervous system."

CWD bacteria (also known as L-forms) can revert to the classical form of a bacteria with a rigid cell wall. When cultured in a petri dish with an antibiotic that destroys cell walls, they will shed their cell wall and revert to the classical L-form.

Human cells have fluid membranes – not rigid cell walls – hence antibiotics like Penicillin that destroy cell walls do not harm human cells. Bacteria with cell walls are therefore vulnerable to antibiotic drugs. The cell wall is also readily identified by white blood cells that consume and destroy them. Under a microscope, when the cell wall is "shed", the bacteria escapes antibiosis as well as attack by the immune system.

CWD bacteria are like criminals using a disguise to hide from the police to enjoy a serial cell-killing spree. ***Their disguise is almost bullet proof because without a cell wall they are essentially invisible.*** Even the blood-brain barrier can be crossed, resulting in a host of neuromuscular disorders in the host. Predictably, ALS-like symptoms have been repeatedly connected to CWD Mycoplasma infections:

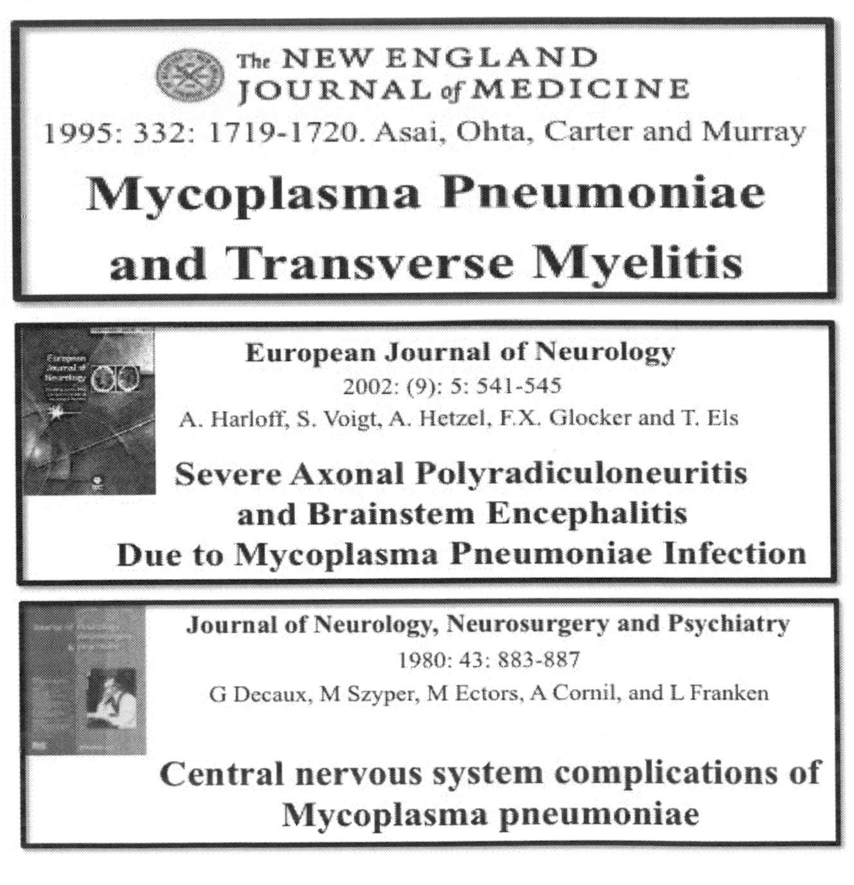
The NEW ENGLAND JOURNAL of MEDICINE
1995: 332: 1719-1720. Asai, Ohta, Carter and Murray
Mycoplasma Pneumoniae and Transverse Myelitis

European Journal of Neurology
2002: (9): 5: 541-545
A. Harloff, S. Voigt, A. Hetzel, F.X. Glocker and T. Els
Severe Axonal Polyradiculoneuritis and Brainstem Encephalitis Due to Mycoplasma Pneumoniae Infection

Journal of Neurology, Neurosurgery and Psychiatry
1980: 43: 883-887
G Decaux, M Szyper, M Ectors, A Cornil, and L Franken
Central nervous system complications of Mycoplasma pneumoniae

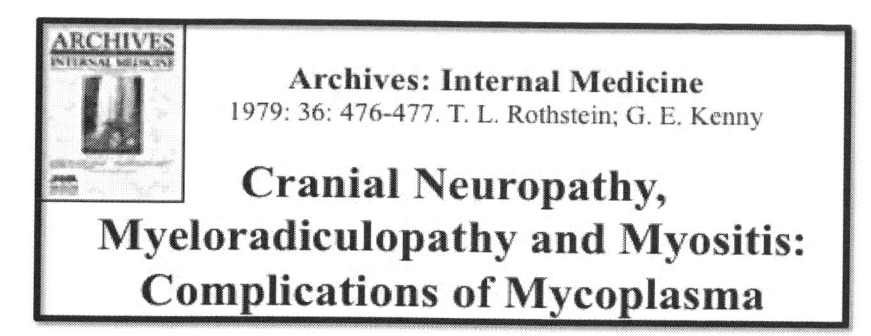

Archives: Internal Medicine
1979: 36: 476-477. T. L. Rothstein; G. E. Kenny

Cranial Neuropathy, Myeloradiculopathy and Myositis: Complications of Mycoplasma

Since penicillin was first discovered by accident in 1928, almost a century has passed for bacteria to mutate and resist these drugs. Most antibiotics like penicillin are, after all, fungal toxins. These toxins are made and employed by fungi to kill competing fungi and other single-celled microbes. Nature accommodates the fittest that survive the germ warfare.

Who are we to think that by ingesting these fungal toxins and calling it "good", that the same does not happen to the microbes that normally live in balance within us? Since nature is hard wired to recombine genes to survive environmental insults, why would not our normal friendly bacteria do the same to combat mycotoxins regularly employed against them?

We make much to-do about proven antibiotic resistance with disease-causing bacteria. *What about our friendly bacteria?*

Are we nuts? Or does fear of death and disease – and ultimately love of money – make us do nutty things like make more, sell more, buy more and consume more toxic drugs – that make more diseases to which we ascribe more scary sounding names to make more drugs to ingest and so the spin goes.

And so it is that many CWD bacteria can be man-made by culturing classical bacteria with antibiotics like the "miracle drug" penicillin. We can stand amazed and watch bacteria under a microscope shed their "coat" and yet survive in their membranous "skin" that is fluid like human white blood cell (macrophage) membranes. In time, they can remake their protein coat – and then take it off again – and on again – and off again.

These CWD microbes seem to say to us, “Na, na, na, na, na, na; now you see me, now you don't!”

Are some of the disease-causing CWD bacteria the result of antibiotic resistance? That man is at least partly to blame for these cell serial killers is obvious. Whether or not some or all of them represent new drug-resistant pathogens, the true serial killers remain the self-appointed pharisees of medicine as long they continue to ignore these infectious microbes and mollify the horrific pain that they cause by prescribing cytotoxic drugs, dismissing the evidence and sending the suffering on their way without a second thought.

“Sorry; we only have 15 minutes. Try this. Next patient, please!”

Bottom Line: Current medical treatment regimens for ALS are based upon a theory that a confused immune system needs to be suppressed by toxic drugs. The possibility of a real infection that needs extermination is either missed or ignored.

Chapter 9: Beware the Yeast

"Beware the yeast of the pharisees."
-Yashua of Nazareth

Less is known about CWD bacteria than is known. They are extremely difficult to culture. It takes a special microscope using live fluid and tissue samples to see them which is not used. The most powerful microscopes commonly used today – the electron microscope – kills the microbes. This makes it very difficult for them to even be seen, and impossible to study their life cycles.

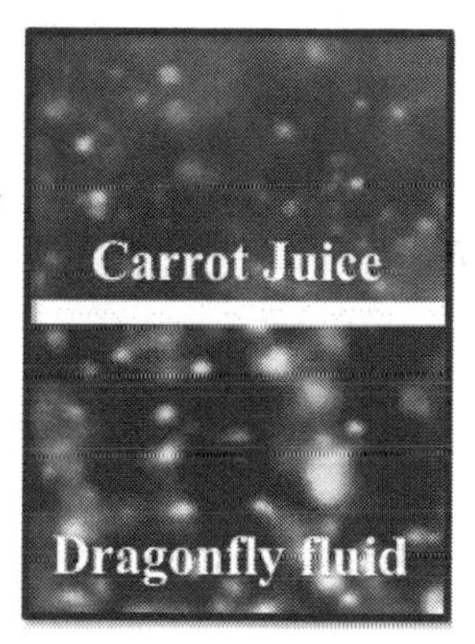

With a somatoscope (developed by Gaston Naessens of Canada), CWD bacteria are magnified with condensed light so that they can be seen in real-time. Naessens calls normal Mycoplasma "somatids" – found in all humans, animals, insects and plants. With the somatoscope, they light up and bounce around in blood, lymph fluid or fresh plant juice like tiny "dancing" particles of light!

Most physicians are completely unaware that Mycoplasma are normally found in blood and fluids of all forms of life. They can not be seen with routine microscopy using dead cell samples. They slip through urine analysis machines undetected. When they

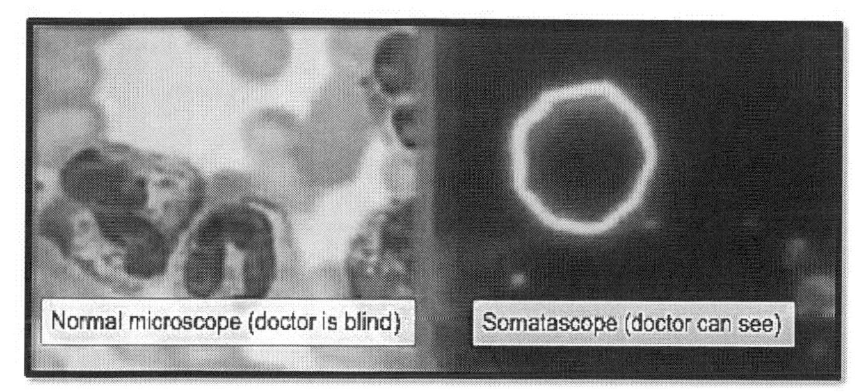

infect the urinary tract system – and they often do – a urine test will often be positive for elevated white blood cells but negative for bacteria. This result is incongruent with conventional medical thinking because normal urine is sterile; there should be no bacteria AND no white blood cells. Most physicians will quickly dismiss the slightly "off" results as due to a "dirty catch".

Not knowing about Mycoplasma is like taking apart an engine, ignoring the rod caps, reassembling the engine and declaring it will work better than ever. It is arrogance mingled with ignorance of the highest order. Beware the yeast of the pharisees.

Mycoplasma pneumoniae was first identified in 1898 at the Pasteur Institute. It was later called "Mycoplasma" because it is fungal-like ("myco") with a fluid membrane that changes shape ("plasma") like a macrophage. This is different than typical fungi with rigid cell walls. They are a kingdom unto themselves – called "mollicutes" – Latin for "soft skin".

Like fungi, under some environmental conditions Mycoplasma change to a form with a rigid cell wall. Like typical fungi, within the rigid cells wall are spores. Like typical fungi, Mycoplasma transit through a life cycle with both sexual reproduction (spore formation) and asexual reproduction (budding).

In the entire kingdom of fungi, about 1% (1,500 species) are yeast. Yeast are single cells that reproduce asexually by asymmetrical division; this is called "budding". Like yeast, Mycoplasma divide by budding; this can be seen real-time in normal human blood Mycoplasma using a somatoscope:

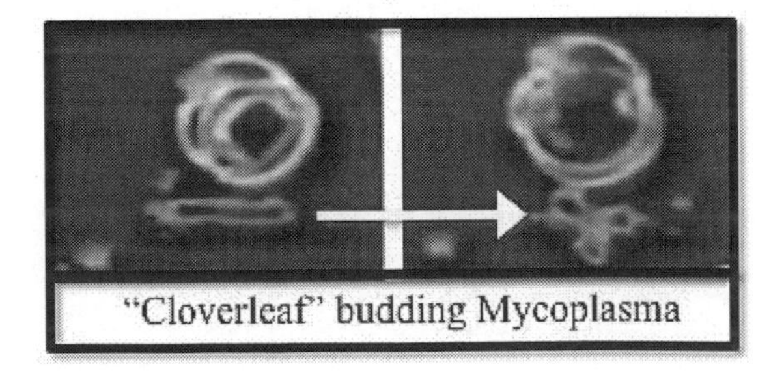
"Cloverleaf" budding Mycoplasma

There are three kingdom of bacteria:

1. Gram positive ("Firmacutes" with firm cell walls)
2. Gram negative ("Gracilicutes" with thin cell walls)
3. Mollicutes (no cell walls)

Physicians spend much time studying the first two – and little to no time learning about the third. As a result, little is widely known about the mollicutes.

Physicians are taught that bacteria do not change form; infectious diseases are "cookie cut" into cause and effect of the disease causing bacteria that have "cookie cut" rigid cell walls. But what about the at-times not-so-cute mollicutes? Not only do they change shapes – but they sometimes take on a rigid cell wall, sometimes behave like fungi, and sometimes take on a rod-shape typical of some firmacutes and gracilicutes and then change back into a round shape and bud like yeast!

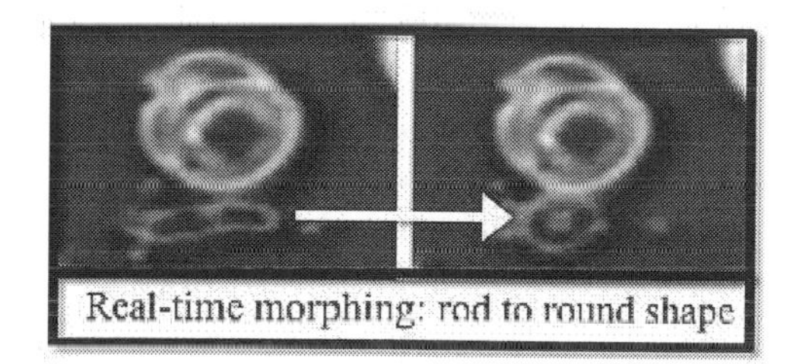
Real-time morphing: rod to round shape

A video of all of this is found at the following on-line link: http://www.youtube.com/watch?v=Py-hutc5ZNM. Watch for yourselves – they are fascinating!

Like mycoplasma, yeasts are single cells, although some species of yeast may become multicellular like fungi by forming a string of budding cells known as pseudohyphae (false hyphae). This is also seen in molds.

So here we have an organism that can live with or without a cell wall, divide asexually by budding, has spores like yeast and creates complex rigid cell wall true hyphae (filaments) like fungi.

Naessens has videographed the life cycle of the Mycoplasma. In blood, they do not change much but in certain environments, such as blood from people with autoimmune illnesses, they cycle through up to 18 forms like spores, bacteria, mycobacteria, yeast and fungi. This rather complex life cycle leaves no room to "cookie cut" the diseases they may cause which are, instead, a spectrum that reflects their wide spectrum of behavior. Here is a simplified version of Naessens' repeated observations:

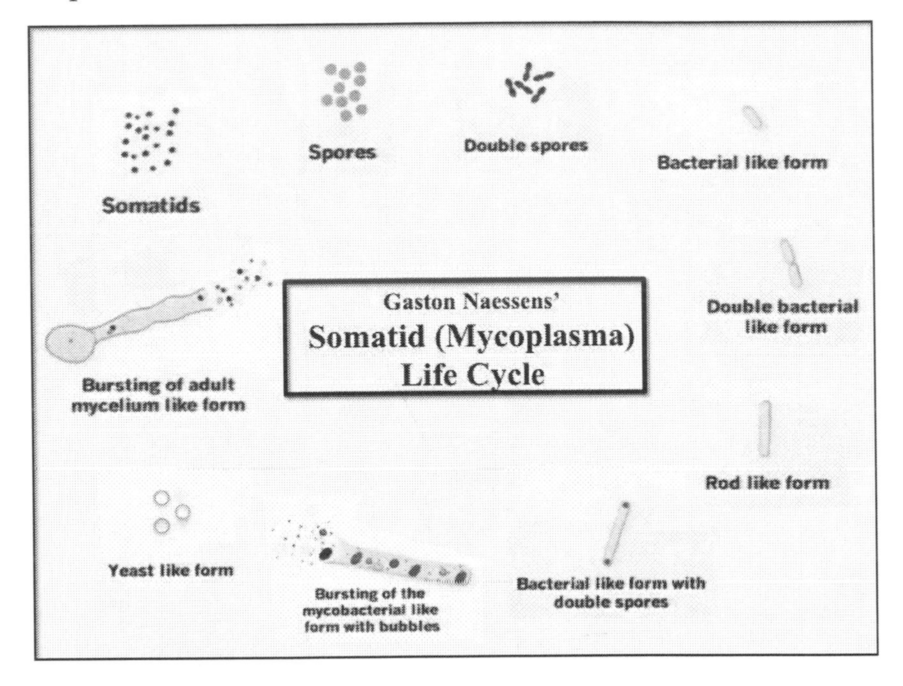

The mycelium (hyphae or firm filaments) that Mycoplasma form are indisputably like a fungus. The releasing of spores is also typical of a fungus.

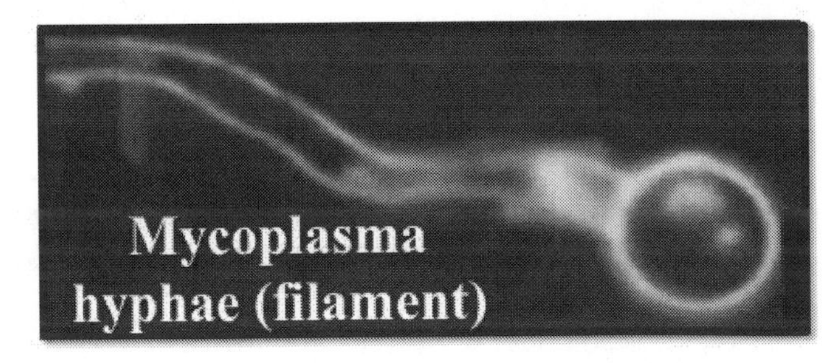

The life cycle of Mycoplasma is remarkably similar to that of dimorphic yeast – the form of which is based upon environmental conditions (oxygen, temperature and nutrients):

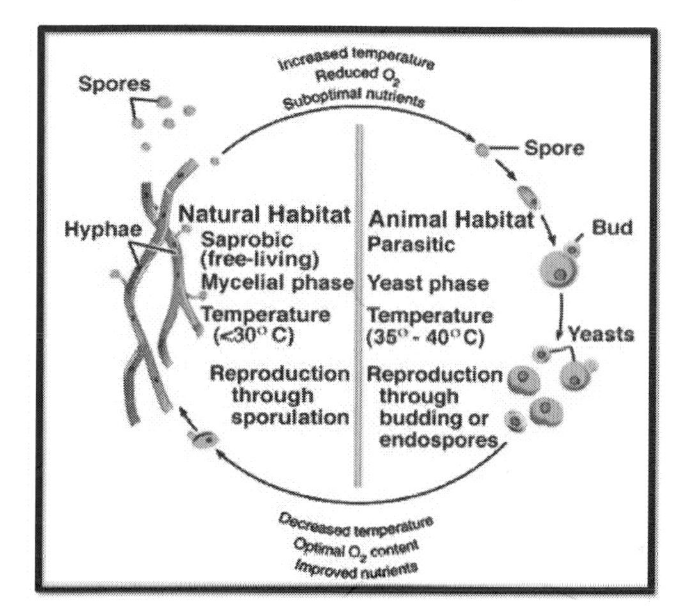

In an acid (low oxygen) terrain, Naessens has observed that the life cycle of Mycoplasma advances past the third or fourth stage into the yeast and mold-like forms. Acidity mimics death; after death, we mold and decay. What turns us to dust when we die?

Did you ever wonder how it is a human body can decay when sealed in a tight casket? *We decay from the inside out.* Mummification slows or prevents this process by killing the Mycoplasma.

We see the same thing with fruit, for example, that becomes overly ripe and too acidic: rot (mold and decay) happens from the inside out. Refrigeration inhibits the Mycoplasma so that fruits and vegetables stay edible a bit longer.

Degenerative disease is a sign of death and decay at the cell, tissue and organ levels. There is no need to turn to mold sooner than later! Likewise, there is no need to ingest dangerous designer drugs to ease the pain of a slow and painful death! A more sensible answer is to maintain your body water in a pH range that keeps Mycoplasma your friends and not your foes.

Normal blood Mycoplasma observed with a somatoscope will routinely congregate around the membranes of white and red blood cells. They behave like "garbage pickers" – cleaning up the membranes. Like tiny fish that clean sharks' teeth, the relationship appears to be symbiotic.

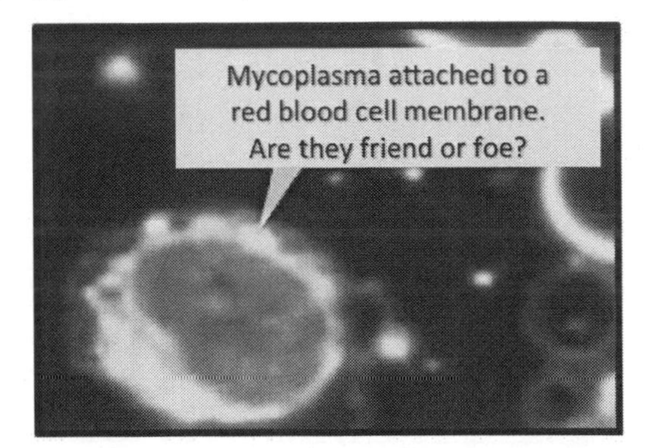

Are they friend or foe? Your doctor does not know! The most sensible answer yet awaiting scientific exploration and substantiation is: "It depends." In an acidic environment, we know they morph into fungal and yeast-like organisms. Since the advent of soft drinks, which are 10,000 more acidic than human blood, anemias and leukemias have been on the rise. Chronic anemias and leukemias have all been associated with chronic infections of pathogenic mollicutes. It is neither kind nor loving to serve the people you love metal cleaner to drink!

Dead oxidized Mycoplasma and cholesterol fill the plaques of diseased heart vessels and arteries; this is called cardiovascular disease or CVD. CVD only occurs in arteries and not veins. Notably, oxidizing fluids that are drunk on an empty stomach are absorbed through the stomach and small intestinal walls *directly into the arteries and not veins*. Soda and chlorinated water drunk on an empty stomach are a direct assault on membranes that line the arteries and are dissolved in the blood.

Chlorine is added to public water supplies because it quickly kills microbes by destroying (oxidizing) the outer cell walls and membranes. What does it do, then, to the Mycoplasmas that are part of normal blood? What does it do to the dietary fats and lipids, like cholesterol, that are part of normal cell and mollicute membranes and are also dissolved in the blood?

We think we're so smart! And because humans are so resistant to change, it may take centuries to alter current ways of thinking and doing business – *even if it kill us*.

New advances in lab techniques – called "PCR" – have enhanced the ability to detect the presence of various strains of Mycoplasma in lab samples. In the last twenty years, other disease causing species of Mycoplasma have been identified. While Mycoplasma pneumoniae typically attaches to the outside of cells, these newly identified mollicutes have lost their genes for amino acid and fatty acid synthesis, forcing them to invade and steal proteins and isoprenoids from healthy cells to survive.

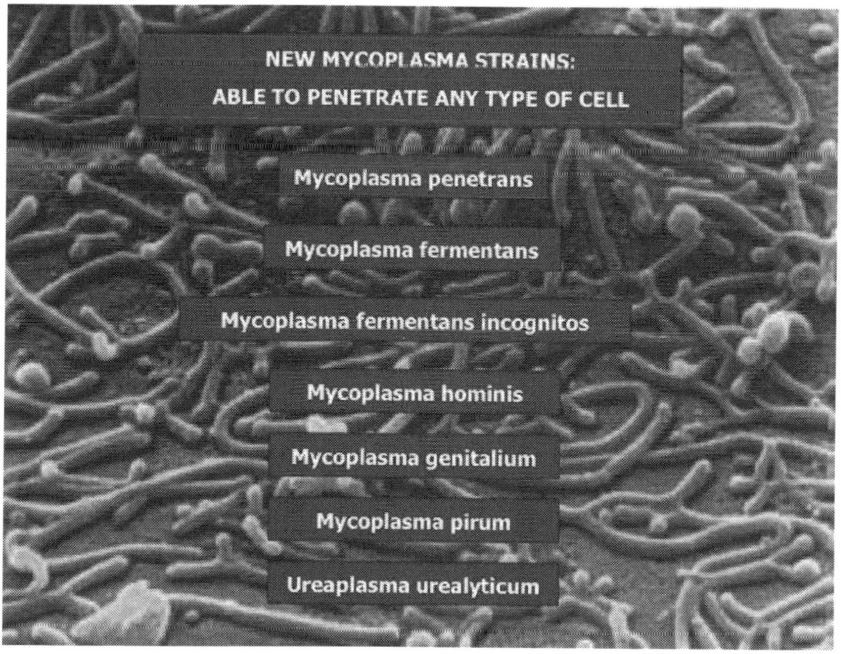

These Mycoplasma are able to penetrate any type of cell.

When Mycoplasma take on the filamentous form, they look just like fungi, The photo below and on page 51 were both taken with scanning electron microscopes:

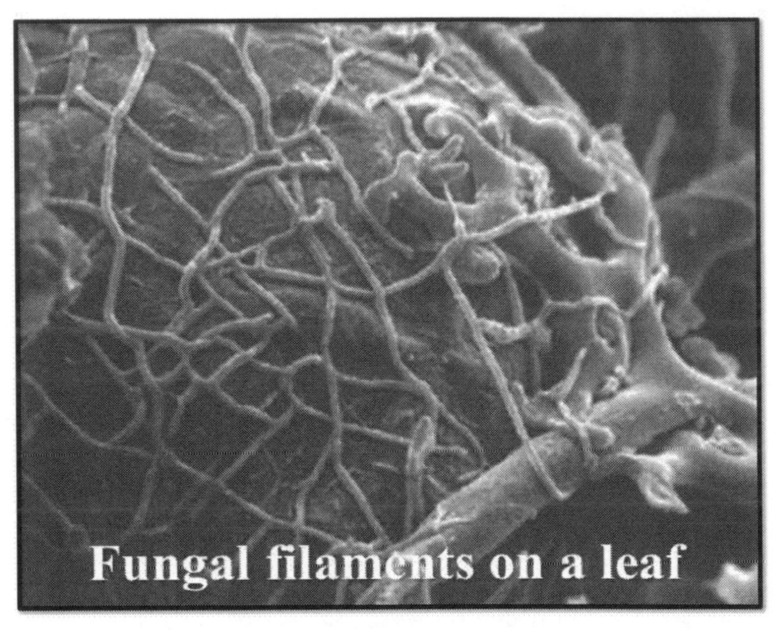

Again, below is Mycoplasma from a human blood sample (see any similarities with the above filament forming fungi?):

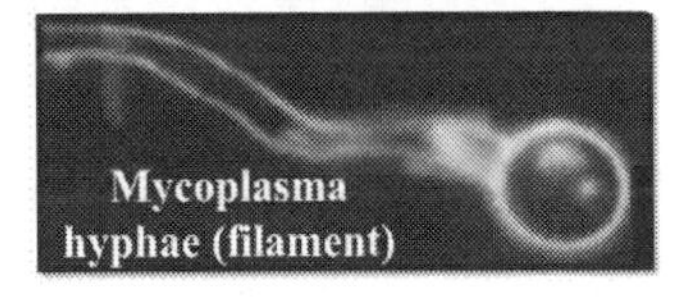

Although some Mycoplasmas belong to the normal flora, many species are pathogens, causing various diseases that tend to run a chronic course. They have been linked to central nervous system disorders and inflammation of the liver, muscle, blood vessels, blood cells, heart and kidneys – and cancer.

The connection of Mycoplasmas to various illnesses such as autoimmune disease is not unlike the connection ultimately made between Helicobacter pylori and stomach ulcers. Helicobacter pylori is not easy to eradicate because it, too, sheds its coat and takes on a CWD form! It, too, loves an acid swimming pool and hides in the cells of the stomach. Because it, too, is a shape shifter, a combined regimen of antibiotics and bismuth must be used to root it out of the stomach and small intestines.

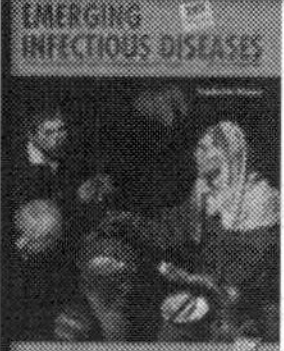

EMERGING INFECTIOUS DISEASES

Center for Disease Control 1998: 4 (3)

Gail H. Cassell. Lilly Research Laboratories, Indianapolis, Indiana, USA

Infectious Causes of Chronic Inflammatory Diseases and Cancer

"One well-known example is the discovery that stomach ulcers are due to *Helicobacter pylori*...A number of infectious agents that cause or contribute to neoplastic diseases in humans have been documented in the past six years. The association and causal role of infectious agents in chronic inflammatory diseases and cancer have major implications for public health, treatment, and prevention."

The scientific database is replete with case reports that connect a wide spectrum of chronic diseases with Mycoplasmas:

Mycoplasma genitalium	Arthritis, nongonococcal urethritis, Pelvic Inflammatory Disease (PID), urogenital infections, infertility
Mycoplasma fermentans	Arthritis, Fibromyalgia, Chronic Fatigue Syndrome, Lupus, autoimmune diseases, ALS, Psoriasis, Scleroderma, Crohn's disease, Irritable Bowel Syndrome, cancer, endocrine disorders, Multiple Sclerosis, Diabetes,
Mycoplasma salivarium	Arthritis, TMJ disorders, eye/ear infections, periodontal/gum disease
Mycoplasma hominis Ureaplasma urealyticum	PID, urogenital infections, prostatitis, epididymitis, urethritis, nephritis, renovascular hypertension, infertility, vaginitis, cervicitis, amnionitis, pyelonephritis, neonatal pneumonia, conjunctivitis, Reiter's syndrome, peritonitis
Mycoplasma pneumoniae	Pneumonia, asthma, respiratory diseases, heart diseases, leukemia, Steven-Johnson syndrome, Crohn's disease, Irritable Bowel Syndrome, arthritis, myositis, tendonitis, polyradiculitis, CNS disorders, Guillain-Barre syndrome, Multiple Sclerosis, Raynaud's phenomenon, restless leg syndrome, hemolytic anemia, transverse myelitis, stroke, hepatitis, encephalitis, meningitis, CFS, myeloradiculopathy, rhabdomyolysis, renal failure, recurrent tonsillitis, recurrent otitis, vasculitis, antiphospholipid syndrome, fibromyalgia
Mycoplasma fermentans (incognitus)	AIDS/HIV, Gulf War Syndrome, autoimmune diseases

Evidence, that can no longer be ignored, supports a more sensible paradigm that "autoimmune" illnesses are *normal* immune responses to one or more undetected CWD pathogens hiding inside cells. And because CWD microbes can infect any cell type, the list of scary sounding diseases they induce is exhaustive.

In the following chapter, the toxins made by some fungi and CWD bacteria is discussed. These toxins – called mycotoxins – can cause cell death by a process called *apoptosis*. When this happens in cells that line the stomach it leaves "scars" called ulcers. ***When this happens in the glial cells that line nerves – it leaves multiple scars – called Amyotrophic Lateral Sclerosis.***

Once identified, Mycoplasmas are treatable with well accepted modalities. To not test and treat for infectious Mycoplasmas is to allow a smoldering infection to cause potentially debilitating permanent tissue damage and/or to be communicated to other persons – as in the well documented STDs of Mycoplasma genitalium. For a physician to so do is to violate the overarching mandate to do no harm and prevent, detect and treat infectious disease.

THE PATHOGENESIS AND TREATMENT OF MYCOPLASMAL INFECTIONS

Antimicrobics and Infectious Disease Newsletter
Elsevier Science1999
Nicolson and Nasralla

"Pathogenic mycoplasmas have been found in the blood or other specimens of patients with a variety of chronic clinical conditions, including…autoimmune, inflammatory and immunosuppressive diseases and fatigue syndromes of unknown origin."

If you want to make some real change in helping to advance proven cures for autoimmune illnesses like ALS, start with a trip to Canada and see Gaston Naesson's magnificent somatoscope for yourself. Who knows; you might even enjoy the opportunity to meet the gentle genius while he's still alive (in his 80's). Then, stop marching for all the foundations supposedly searching for cures that are never going to be found. The people who run those businesses have no incentive but to forever wear blinders, even if answers are clearly put right before their eyes. Finally, lobby your local school boards and put somatoscopes in high schools – ***because the pharisees don't want to see the yeast***.

The pharisees don't want to see the yeast because if they do, they lose their control over their patients – and a whole lot of money. It is time for medicine to reject its current dark age, turn on somatoscopes en masse, light up the mollicutes and sort it all out.

Bottom Line: Human blood and fluids in all living things contain the tiniest lifeforms on earth and which may yet prove to be the "essence" of all life – and chronic disease and death. Mollicutes change into various forms, depending on pH, temperature, oxygen and nutrients. Less is known about them than is known. While they support life they are clearly involved in chronic degenerative, inflammatory and autoimmune diseases. Time is long overdue for somatoscopes to be delivered to our youth because the old pharisees are not giving way to the truth that sets men free.

Chapter 10: Cereal Killers

"I am convinced digestion is the great secret to life."
-Sydney Smith

By the early 1980's, physicians still believed that stomach ulcers were caused by too much as acid in the stomach from stress or spicy food. Even though treatment with milk diets and acid blockers offered some relief, symptoms frequently recurred.

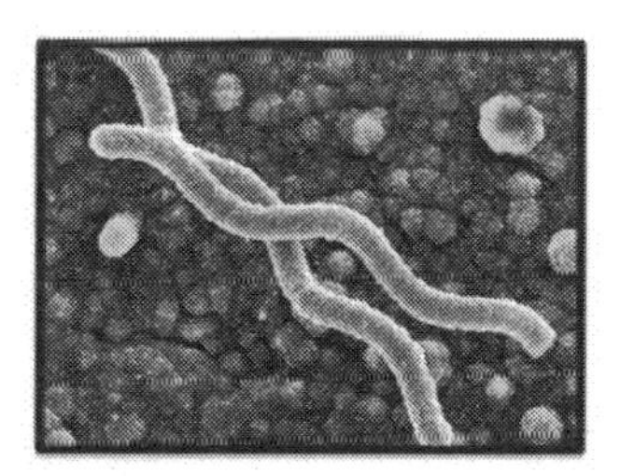

In 1982, Drs. Marshall and Warren of Perth, Australia presented evidence that there was a connection between over-proliferation of acid-loving spiral shaped "H. pylori" bacteria in the stomach. These had been discovered almost a century earlier in dogs and are found in the stomach of many healthy people. But Marshall and Warren believed that over-proliferation of these bacteria could cause gastritis, ulcers and stomach cancer. They presented their finds, but skeptics turned a deaf ear and insisted the microbes were innocent bystanders.

Marshall grew tired of the naysayers and by 1985 it was time to put an end to it. He drank a flask of cultured H. pylori and gave himself a bad case of gastritis. He recovered, and within a few short years physicians were finally eradicating ulcers with antibiotics and bismuth. Ten years later, Marshall and Warren shared a Nobel prize.

H. pylori frequently takes on a CWD form (reference 22). While I am absolutely convinced that dozens of other pathogenic CWD bacteria are the ultimate source of many other "autoimmune" inflammatory diseases, I am not about to drink a flask of them. Crazy Aussie; I am proud of him! He deserves more than a Nobel for having so quickly changed the minds of so many men!

In the Louvre hangs a famous 16th century painting called "The Beggars" by Pieter Bruegel the Elder. It remains shrouded in mystery as to the meaning of the foxtails that hang from capes worn by the beggars

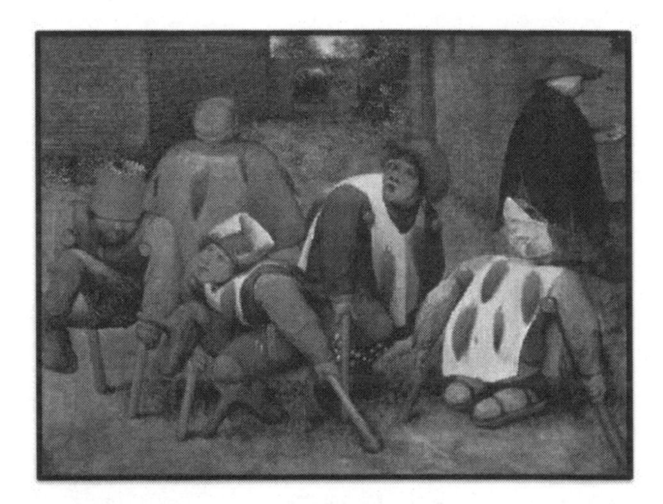

I suggest the beggars were victims of foxtail poisoning or ergotism – epidemic in the Netherlands during medieval times. The foxtail ponchos were probably distinctive clothing like leper's capes. It is a heart-rending possibility that the fools' caps further tagged these poor souls, who suffered loss of mentation as well as limb, as public laughing stocks.

Foxtail millet, the oldest cultivated gluten-free cereal grain, is native to Bruegel's home in the wet, lowlands of the Netherlands. Ergotism is caused by ingesting a mycotoxin from a parasitic fungus that infests edible grass grains like the foxtail grown in excessively damp conditions.

Victims of ergotism suffered from burning sensations, swollen legs due to loss of circulation, gangrene and finally below-the-knee amputations. Today, these same complications plague victims with type 2 diabetes.

Mycotoxins (fungal toxins) like the ergot frequently infect grains and can be vicious cereal killers. Likewise, toxins from at times fungal-like CWD bacteria can be vicious serial killers. A preponderance of evidence supports that *toxins* are the link between inflammation syndromes of H. pylori (gastritis, etc.) and the various inflammatory conditions associated with autoimmune diseases (myositis, neuritis, uveitis, hepatitis, etc.).

H. pylori is difficult to both detect and treat because it can convert to a round CWD form ("Na, na, na, na, na, na..."). As a result, combination antibiotics only achieve 75 to 90% eradication rates – not bad, but not sure-fire.

Probiotics, on the other hand, are proving more effective than antibiotics at countering the destructive effects of H. pylori (references 23 and 24). This smoking gun points to ulcers by H. pylori infection as due to an imbalance of normal gut flora and over proliferation of H. pylori and its toxins. And, since antibiotics do not completely eradicate the "now you see me now you don't" CWD forms of H. pylori that invade cells and cause immune dysfunction (reference 22), it seems CWD H. pylori variants are yet tamed by some probiotics (normal gut flora).

H. pylori toxins kill cells that line the stomach and duodenum by apoptosis which causes inflammation and ultimately ulcers. *Ulcers are inflamed pits or scars not unlike that seen in myelin with ALS* (references 25 and 26). Cell death can occur in two ways: necrosis (normal cell death) or apoptosis ("genotoxicity" or death by DNA destruction). H. pylori toxins, like fungal toxins or mycotoxins, kill cells by apoptosis.

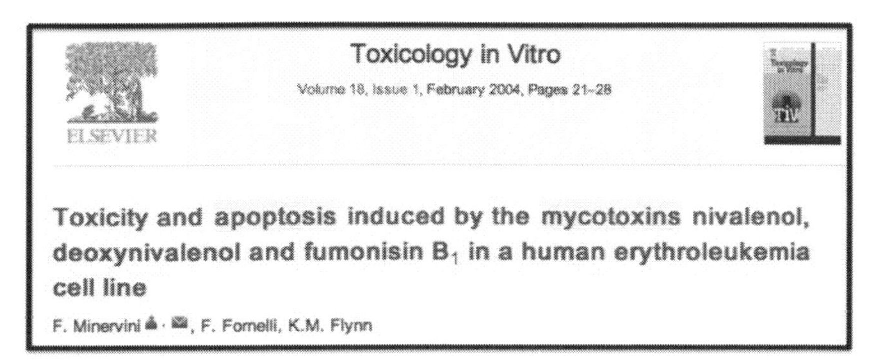
ELSEVIER

Toxicology in Vitro

Volume 18, Issue 1, February 2004, Pages 21–28

Toxicity and apoptosis induced by the mycotoxins nivalenol, deoxynivalenol and fumonisin B_1 in a human erythroleukemia cell line

F. Minervini, F. Fornelli, K.M. Flynn

Mycotoxins are “secondary metabolites” made by disease causing fungi. All cells and most all microbes make primary metabolites that are essential to life. Secondary metabolites are toxins made by some poisonous fungi, like the species that causes foxtail poisoning. ***These toxins mimic primary metabolites.***

In the cutthroat world of filamentous fungi, mycotoxins mimic primary metabolites. If a fungus competes for valuable real estate, it can make a toxic secondary metabolite that looks, smells and tastes like a primary metabolite. It's a more clever strategy than directly assaulting an “enemy” with a poison, only to have it “sniff out” and evade the bait. Mycotoxins mimic “good food”. If a single-celled competing microbe is fooled and ingests the deadly toxin, the mycotoxin-making fungus keeps the turf. In multi-celled mammals, many mycotoxins lower blood cholesterol by a series of reactions by cells made to overcome death by apoptosis. An example are statin drugs that lower blood cholesterol; these are mycotoxins extracted from filamentous fungi:

Bonn 2010

Analysis of the genetic potential of the sponge-derived fungus *Penicillium chrysogenum* E01-10/3 for polyketide production

Fungal mycotoxins

Mycotoxins are known as low-molecular-weight natural products (i.e. small molecules) produced as secondary metabolites in filamentous fungi. These metabolites represent a chemically heterogeneous group, but they all exhibit high toxicity. By definition mycotoxins are synthesised in filamentous fungi and are toxic to vertebrates and other animal groups in extremely low (i.e. microgram) concentrations [15]. When present in food, these fungal metabolites can have toxic effects with acute (e.g. liver or kidney deterioration) and chronic (e.g. liver cancer) symptoms. Due to their mutagenic and teratogenic profile, exposure to fungal metabolites may result in skin irritation, immunosuppression, birth defects, neurotoxicity and death [16]

The members of the statin family of secondary metabolites are potent inhibitors of 3-hydroxy-3-methylglutaryl-coenzyme A (HMG-CoA) reductase, the key enzyme in cholesterol biosynthesis in humans [87].

There are many ways to lower cholesterol. Some snake venoms will do the trick. If you're willing to take the risk, so will a few poisonous mycotoxins from common blue-green food molds. If you've been taking statin drugs, you've already indulged. These common mycotoxins are from Aspergillus and Penicillium fungi that commonly infest corn, nuts and grains:

- Aflatoxin
- Citrinin
- Fumonisins
- Luteoskyrin
- Ochratoxin-A
- Patulin
- Rubratoxin-B
- Statin (Monocolin K)
- Zearalenone

Aspergillus and Penicillium fungi readily contaminate grains growing in wet fields or stored in damp silos. They are easy to identify because they have a lactone ring that fluoresces under UV light. The lactone ring mimics the portion of an enzyme that competing microbes and human cells need to make isoprenoids. The lactone ring can be deadly (reference 35).

Isoprenoids support cell functions such as metabolism, replication and membrane stability. Most CWD bacteria have lost the ability to make vital isoprenoids so they enter cells or single-celled microbes and rob them from the host. The lactose ring in many mycotoxins mimics an enzyme called “reductase” that competing fungi and microbes (and human cells) use to make isoprenoids to grow and replicate. ***Poisonous fungi make them to mimic primary metabolites and kill competing organisms.***

Because isoprenoids give membranes strength (dolichol and cholesterol), make energy (CoQ10) and promote DNA and cell replication (isopentenyl adenine), when isoprenoid synthesis is blocked by a mycotoxin the DNA falls apart and the cell or single-celled microbe dies by apoptosis. In multi-celled mammals, isoprenoid levels such as cholesterol drop in the blood. Blood cholesterol levels are lowered at the expense of killing cells in organs and tissues by apoptosis!

[CANCER RESEARCH 51, 3602-3609, July 1, 1991]

Synchronization of Tumor and Normal Cells from G_1 to Multiple Cell Cycles by Lovastatin[1]

Khandan Keyomarsi,[2] Larue Sandoval, Vimla Band, and Arthur B. Pardee

Divisions of Cell Growth and Regulation [K. K., L. S., A. B. P.] and Cancer Genetics [V. B.], Dana Farber Cancer Institute, Boston, Massachusetts 02115

In this paper, we report that these criteria for synchronization are met using Lovastatin to arrest normal and tumor cells of epithelial as well as fibroblast origin reversibly in the G_1 phase of the cell cycle. Lovastatin, an antihyperlipodemic agent, is widely used for the treatment of hypercholesterolemia. This agent competitively inhibits HMG-CoA[3] reductase, the enzyme required for conversion of HMG-CoA to mevalonic acid (8). In addition, inhibition of mevalonate synthesis by Lovastatin or compactin, a related fungal toxin (9), also inhibits DNA replication (10–15). DNA replication is restored by the addition of mevalonate, the product of the reaction catalyzed by HMG-CoA reductase.

Human cells that die by apoptosis induced by a mycotoxin leave behind pits, ulcers and scars. If this happens to stomach cells, we see ulcers. If this happens to glial cells that make myelin, "multiple scars"are visualized on MRI scans. If this happens to red blood cells, it causes hemolytic anemia.

Apoptotic activity induced by the mycotoxins ochratoxin A and zearalenone in bovine lymphocytes

M.B. Lioi[1], A. Santoro[1], R. Barbieri[1], S. Salzano[2], M.V. Ursini[3]

ITAL.J.ANIM.SCI. VOL. 2 (SUPPL. 1), 94-96, 2003

Many mycotoxins are neurotoxic. Fumonisins, penetrems and territrems, for example, are universally present in peanuts, corn and wheat products. These can cause tremors, convulsions, limb weakness, and ataxis (unsteady gait) – not unlike symptoms of ALS.

Most physicians would diagnose mycotoxicity and resultant tissue damage by apoptosis (causing spasms and shakes) as one or more of the following:

1. Amyotrophic Lateral Sclerosis (a nerve destroying muscle wasting condition).
2. Parkinson's disease (a very shaky muscular condition).
3. MS (another very nerve scarring muscular condition).

Because of the broad spectrum of symptoms caused by different toxins, there are often as many different diagnoses as there are different physician consultations. What different MD's would most likely agree upon, nevertheless, is that the neuromuscular trouble would be attributed to some "genetic proclivity" rather than possible mycotoxicity from a common food mold. Much of the hub-bub about genetics and disease is a smokescreen to "baffle the commoners with BS". This does little more than to preserve composure and the status quo when no one wants to admit that no one knows for sure what the hell is really going on.

It is believed that tissue damage in autoimmune diseases, such as the multiple myelin scars in peripheral nerves with ALS, are due to cell death by the immune system's white blood cells – hence the term "autoimmunity". Found at the scene of the crime are pits and scars and sometimes inflammation (white blood cells).

There is sufficient evidence, on the other hand, to demonstrate that tissue damage in the face of known disease causing CWD, is indirectly due to CWD bacterial toxins and not directly by white blood cells *or even CWD bacteria.*

CWD bacterial toxins, like mycotoxins, destroy cells by apoptosis. This has been documented with H. pylori (references 25 and 26), Chlamydia pneumoniae (references 27-29), Mycoplasma pnemoniae (references 30-32) and many other pathogenic CWD bacteria. ***Various toxins that induce apoptosis have been discovered in these shape-shifting and at time yeast and fungal like CWD bacteria.***

While antibiotic regimens have been recommended by some physicians for CWD infections – this, too, could be a presumptive knee-jerk reaction that addresses symptoms and not root cause. What if some CWD bacteria are the scourge of antibiotic resistance? We have, after all, enjoyed over eight decades of indiscriminate use of antibiotics like penicillin *that work by destroying bacterial cell walls*.

Are the CWD microbes fighting back? Fungal toxins like penicillin that block cell wall production normally do not affect human cells – because human cells do not have cell walls. Microbes are hard-wired to recombine genes so that under the assault of toxins some progeny might survive. The survivors learn to adapt (take off their coat) and/or make their own toxins.

This, rather, is the root of the "genetic proclivity" of chronic degenerative, inflammatory and autoimmune disease! The genes that need to be addressed are not ours – it's our flora ("good" bacteria that normally live in symbiotic balance)!

Are CWD bacteria living examples of proverbial Darwinian "survival of the fittest" strategies to adapt to long-term germ warfare *that we introduced into the human race and our animal food supply in the first place?* Are we too busy, too arrogant, too blind or all of the above to sort it out? Are we going to preserve the definition of "insanity" by trying to achieve different results by doing the same old thing?

I say again: Current treatments for autoimmune diseases do NOT work. Current theories are therefore WRONG.

To not stop the madness is to practice mass malpractice with impunity. There is a good reason why MANY autoimmune diseases are DRUG-INDUCED by a long list of antibiotics and anti-fungals. These include:

- Doxycycline (antibiotic)
- Griseofulvin (antifungal)
- Isoniazid (antibiotic)
- Minocycline (antibiotic)
- Penicillin (antibiotic)
- Pyrazinamide (antibiotic)
- Quinidine (antibiotic)
- Streptomycin (antibiotic)
- Sulfonamides (antibiotic)
- Voriconazole (antifungal)

Many other drugs that induce autoimmune reactions, while not classified as antibiotics, are derived from secondary fungal metabolites and have antibiotic activity. Statins serve as but one example.

I recommend that Pandora's box not be revisited by releasing more antibiotics against microbes that are perhaps releasing their own antibiotics against us. Mycotoxins are, after all, antibiotics (anti-life) and many man-made antibiotics like penicillin are made from mycotoxins in the first place. Has a mycotoxin derived antibiotic resistant kingdom of microbes evolved within us that manufacture their own mycotoxin derived antibiotics against us – only no one noticed because it happened inside human cells? Have some of our once-normal flora become foes instead of friends?

Furthermore, for decades, we have indiscriminately fed antibiotics to dairy cattle who now succumb to autoimmune diseases. While heating milk kills many antibiotic-resistant and undetected CWD microbes, *it does not destroy heat-resistant toxins that pass into milk.*

God only knows what CWD spores and toxins are passed to us through our meat supply – both by CWD toxins and ingestion of mycotoxin contaminated feed.

And then there is chlorinated water – poison served to us, the animals we eat and a direct hit to the "good" Mycoplasma in our blood that hardly anyone knows about. Chlorine is also a direct hit to the "good" LDL cholesterol dissolved in human blood and which is a vital component of the brain and nervous system – especially myelin. LDL cholesterol is more easily oxidized than HDL cholesterol; when destroyed by oxidation,the liver replaces it and levels rise (reference 35). That LDL levels rise does not make it "bad"; oxidizing LDL in the first place is bad.

While CWD bacteria have been isolated in the cerebrospinal fluid of ALS patients, these can be killed by heating the fluid. Even when the CWD bacteria are killed by heat, a resistant toxin called "gliotoxin" remains active in the CSF that can yet destroy glial cells by apoptosis (reference 33).

This same toxin has been isolated from pathogenic Aspergillus fungi (reference 34). The first FDA approved statin developed by Merck (lovastatin) is a mycotoxin extracted from a pathogenic strain of Aspergillus. Predictably, statins have also been associated with drug-induced ALS and many other autoimmune illnesses (reference 35).

Chem. Rev. **2009**, 109, 3909-3990

Chemistry and Biology of Mycotoxins and Related Fungal Metabolites

Table 2. Mycotoxins Produced by *Aspergillus* sp.

fungus	mycotoxin produced
Aspergillus terreus	Territrem A,[25] Citreoviridin, Citrinin (**2**), Gliotoxin (**527**), Patulin (**3**), Terrein, Terreic acid, Terretonin, Itaconic acid, Aspulvinone, Asterric acid, Asterriquinone, butyrolactone I, Emodin (**573**), Geodin, Itaconate, Lovastatin,[26] Questin, Sulochrin, Terrecyclic acid.

Bottom Line: The preponderance of evidence is that nerve degeneration can be induced by drugs like statins, mycotoxins and gliotoxins from CWD bacteria.

Chapter 11: Don't Lose Your Nerve

"Time is a spiral, space is a curve,
I know you get dizzy but don't lose your nerve."
-Anonymous

The common mantra of today is that there is neither a known cause nor cure for ALS. With the current practice of for-profit medicine, there is little incentive to find the cause and cure of any chronic disease that generates long-term cash flow. There is even more incentive to suppress them when found.

Without known cause(s), there can be no remedy. With known cause(s), there is hope for remedy.

A diagnosis, by definition, implies remedy "through knowledge." ALS is a description of nerve and muscle degeneration. *It is not a diagnosis.*

ALS randomly strikes once-healthy people. The condition breeds fear in facing a cruel and seemingly hopeless fate. Destruction of myelin interrupts normal nerve impulses to nerves and muscle and gradually paralyzes the body. The resultant dreaded symptoms surface as muscle weakness, incoordination, slurred speech, difficulty with swallowing, and increasing shortness of breath until mechanical breathing machines are required to extend life. Prescription drugs only help alleviate symptoms and do not reduce the progression of the disease.

Despite all of the negative press that breeds fear and forever sells sickness, there are three apparent and remedial causes for multiple scars in myelin sheaths:

1. CWD bacterial infection (toxins)
2. Mycotoxins
3. Statin drugs (a mycotoxin)

These are not mutually exclusive. All three cause ALS-like symptoms. ***CWD bacteria and mycotoxins are the common thread of ALS.***

It is time to fuel nerve cells with the needed building blocks to make and maintain new myelin.

While most nerve cells are slow to regenerate, glial nerve cells are not. Glial cells make up to 90 percent of the brain and support the entire nervous system. ***Glial nerve cells rapidly replicate when there is injury.*** This is good news for anyone with ALS because glial cells make myelin – and lots of it!

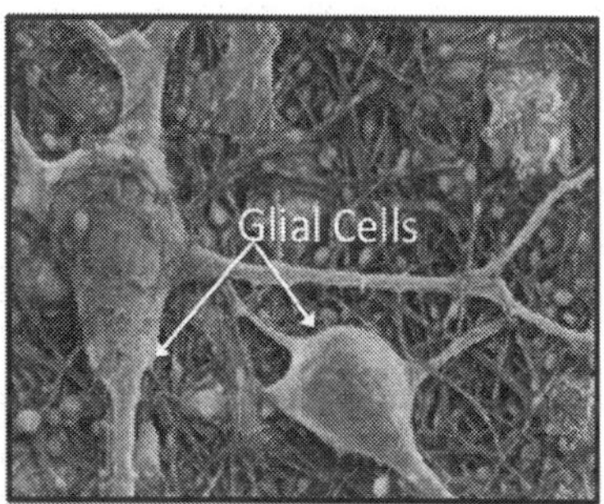

More accurately, glial cells ARE myelin. "Glia" means "glue". Glial cell outgrowths are what make myelin. When glial cells are damaged or destroyed, nerves become "unglued." This leaves scars. If multiple glial cells are destroyed, this leaves nerve and muscle damage – ALS.

Part of supporting glial cells means knowing what to and what not to do. Do not ingest anything that blocks glial cells from making myelin or causes glial cells to become unglued.

For glial cells to maintain or repair myelin, they need to quickly replicate. This is another reason why you do not want to take a statin drug that lowers cholesterol. One of the isoprenoids that statins block cells from making is isopentenyl adenine. This isoprenoid is essential for DNA to replicate.

If DNA is blocked from replicating, glial cells can not replicate. ***Like many mycotoxins and CWD bacteria toxins, statins block glial cell replication and kill glial cells (and muscle cells) by a process called "apoptosis".***

Lovastatin-Induced Proliferation Inhibition and Apoptosis in C6 Glial Cells[1]

JAE W. CHOI and SUNG E. JUNG
Department of Pharmacology, Yonsei University College of Medicine, Seoul, Korea

In this study we demonstrated that the cytotoxic effects of lovastatin fall into two categories: suppression of cell growth and induction of apoptosis of C6 glial cells...In conclusion, our data demonstrate that lovastatin can inhibit cell proliferation and induce apoptosis in C6 glial cells, which highlights the importance of the mevalonate pathway on the regulation of cell proliferation and prevention of apoptosis.

In apoptosis, the normally compact DNA begins to fragment and protrude from the nuclear membrane that houses the DNA. Within 24 hours, glial cell DNA literally falls apart:
Left above: Normal twin-strands of condensed glial cell DNA before lovastatin. Right above: “Ground-zero” after lovastatin. Following fragmentation of the DNA, glial cells die.

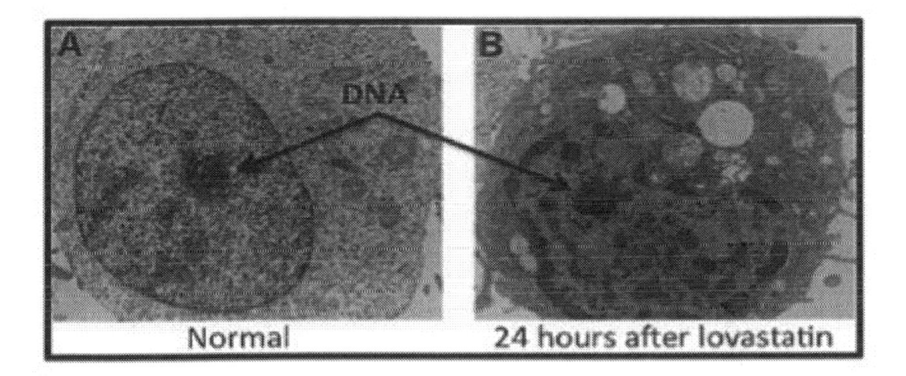

Bottom Line: ***When glial cells die by apoptosis, and are blocked from replicating and therefore replacing myelin, what remains are degenerated nerves. If the nerves are central, the resulting symptoms are more like MS. If the nerves are peripheral, the symptoms are more like ALS.***

Chapter 12: Muscle Matters

"No army can withstand the strength of an idea whose time has come."
-Victor Hugo

In 1960, the term "mycotoxin" was coined after a fungal toxin in commercial nut feed was found as the source of rapid and deadly muscle-wasting cancer epidemics in farm-raised turkey and trout. The discovery spawned the "mycotoxin gold rush" for the next 15 years as drug companies hunted for new toxigenic agents from food molds. As a result, many drugs with antibiotic effects are mycotoxins. They are extracts (ahem, "secondary metabolites" as the drug industry likes to call them) from poisonous fungi.

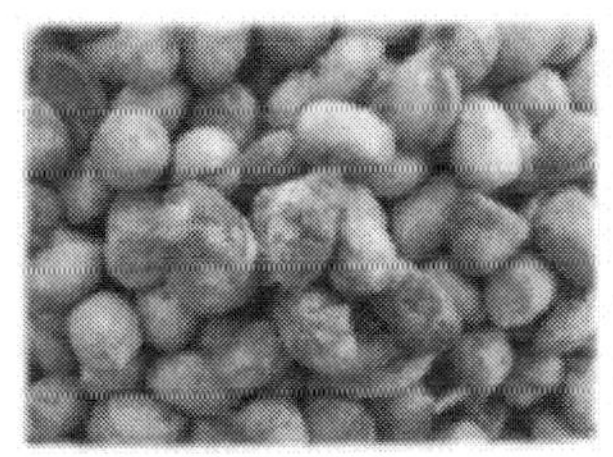

The mycotoxin that caused the 1960 outbreaks of liver cancer was so toxic that it almost decimated the farm-raised rainbow trout population in the U.S. and farm-raised turkey population in the U.K. A new toxin from the blue-green food mold Aspergillus flavus was found to be the cause and given the name "aflatoxin" ("a" from "Aspergillus" and "fla" from "flavus").

The toxicity of aflatoxin is attributed to a specific characteristic of its chemical structure: a polyketide with a lactone ring.

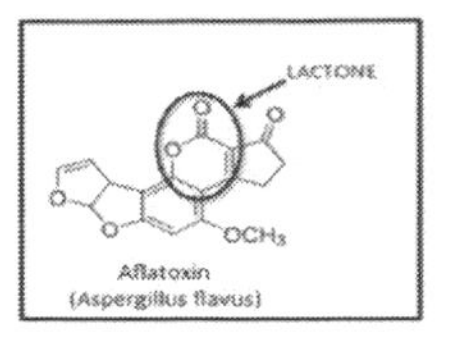

Many polyketide lactone mycotoxins are toxic to nerves and cause tremors; these are called "tremorgenic" toxins. Aspergillus flavus also produces a tremorgenic toxin called "aflatrem". In experimental animals, a single dose of aflatrem causes progressive motor nerve terminal degeneration over a period of weeks; death follows by respiratory failure. These are all ALS related symptoms.

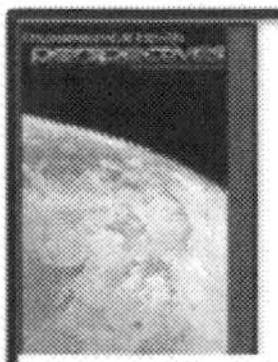

Aflatrem: A Tremorgenic Mycotoxin With Acute Neurotoxic Effecits

Valdes J, Cameron J and Cole R.

"A group of fungal metabolites collectively known as tremorgenic mycotoxins have been identified as the causative agents of a neurological disease of cattle known as "staggers syndrome". This disease is characterized by muscle tremors and hyperexcitability, and similar responses have been observed in laboratory animals treated with the mycotoxins. The fungi which product these compounds have been isolated from corn, silage and various forages, and so pose a health threat for both livestock and humans who consume these commodities."

Environmental Health Perspectives, 1985 (62): 459-63.

The first FDA-approved statin for lowering cholesterol (lovastatin) is also a polyketide mycotoxin with a lactone ring. It is extracted from Aspergillus terreus. Like aflatoxin from Aspergillus flavus, it lowers cholesterol. Like aflatoxin and aflatrem, it causes cancer in experimental animals and induces ALS like symptoms (reference 35).

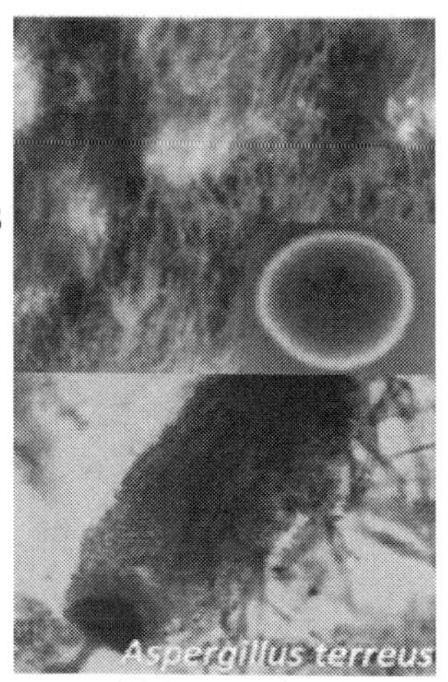

Like Aspergillus flavus, there is nothing good for animals or humans that ever came from Aspergillus terreus – especially statin drugs. Aspergillus terreus is a pathogenic fungus causing aspergillosis, otomycosis, onchomycosis, abscesses of the aorta and various skin infections. Ingestion causes death in rodents and abortions in cattle. Single-celled organisms are simple-fare: it is antibiotic, antifungal and even antiviral against herpes.

Aspergillus terreus mycotoxins are toxic to the kidneys, liver and nervous systems and cause birth defects and cancer. This includes Merck's lovastatin (monocolin-K):

- Citreoviridin
- Citrinin
- Clavacin
- Ferrichrysin
- Geodin
- Monacolin-K (lovastatin)
- Patulin
- Terrecine
- Terretonine
- Territrem-A
- Territrem-B

Chem. Rev. 2009, 109, 3909-3990

Chemistry and Biology of Mycotoxins and Related Fungal Metabolites

Table 2. Mycotoxins Produced by *Aspergillus* sp.

fungus	mycotoxin produced
Aspergillus terreus	Territrem A,[25] Citreoviridin, Citrinin (**2**), Gliotoxin (**527**), Patulin (**3**), Terrein, Terreic acid, Terretonin, Itaconic acid, Aspulvinone, Asterric acid, Asterriquinone, butyrolactone I, Emodin (**573**), Geodin, Itaconate, Lovastatin,[26] Questin, Sulochrin, Terrecyclic acid.

Mycotoxins arc chcmically diverse and range in molecular weight from 200 to 500. Notably, lovastatin ($C_{24}H_{36}O_5$) with a molecular weight of 404.54 grams per mole, is almost identical to citreoviridin ($C_{23}H_{30}O_6$) with a molecular weight of 402.48. In humans, citreoviridin concentrates in the central nervous system and causes an ascending paralysis, convulsions and respiratory arrest (reference 36) – all ALS symptoms. Citreoviridin frequently grows on grain hulls; the first statin was extracted from moldy rice.

In 1979, researchers found that stored rice in Taiwan was heavily polluted by Aspergillus fungi. A family of fungal metabolites was subsequently isolated from chloroform extracts of submerged rice culture of Aspergillus terreus. These fungal metabolites were named “territrem” after Aspergillus “terreus” and the “tremorgenic” activities they induced in lab rats.

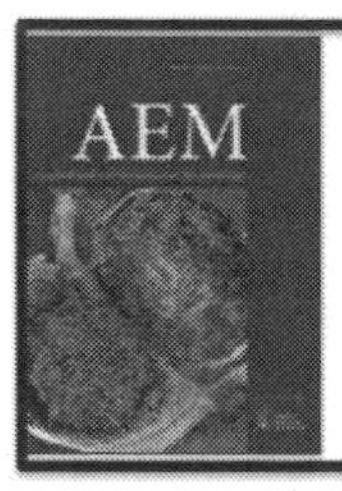

Territrems, Tremorgenic Mycotoxins of Aspergillus terreus

Ling K H, Yang C K and Peng F T.

Applied and Environmental Microbiology, 1979: 37 (3): 355.

Territrem A and B are lactone polyketides with structural similarities to lovastatin (and all other statins for lowering cholesterol). In experimental animals they cause tremors, spasms, twitching and loss of muscle (amyotrophy) – all symptoms of ALS. By a process of exclusion, most physicians would diagnose territrem-induced spasms and shakes as Multiple Sclerosis, Parkinson's or Lou Gehrig's disease. The disease would be attributed to a "genetic proclivity" rather than possible food poisoning by a common grain mold.

More recent work has demonstrated that the territrems are potent poisons that bind irreversibly with an enzyme called acetylcholinesterase that normally degrades the excitatory nerve transmitter acetylcholine. This increases both the level and duration of action of the neurotransmitter acetylcholine – causing tremors and ultimately ALS-like motor nerve degeneration

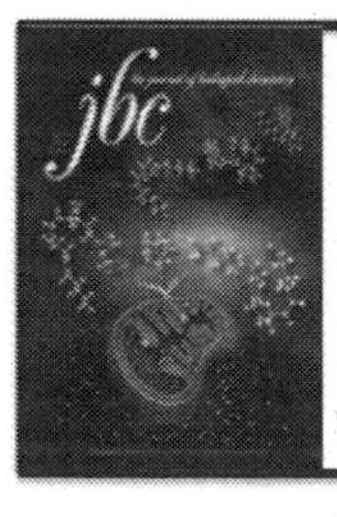

Territrem B, a Tremogenic Mycotoxin That Inhibits Acetylcholinesterase with a Noncovalent yet Irreversible Binding Mechanism

The Journal of Biological Chemistry., 1999: 274 (49): 34916-923

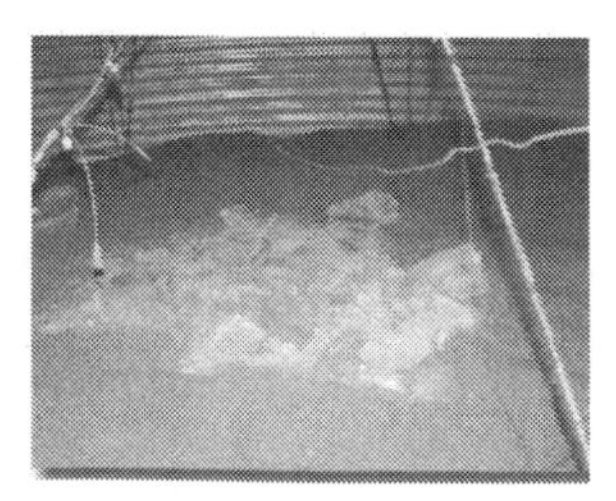

Few if any farmers, upon finding moldy silage, will voluntarily destroy the entire cache. With ingestion of a single common food mold there is risk of multiple *multiple* mycotoxicoses from the same fungus. Mycotoxin poisoning leading to ALS-like symptoms can not be attributed

to a single tremorgenic mycotoxin, because there are *many* toxins from a single pathogenic fungus such as Aspergillus terreus that are neurotoxic. There is an exception to this general rule. Since FDA approval of lovastatin, the effects of a *single* Aspergillus terreus mycotoxin on the nervous system has surfaced. Statins, a single isolated mycotoxin, induce ALS. This same mycotoxin has subsequently been isolated from other pathogenic fungi – hence there are multiple statins sold on the market today that illicit the same ill effects.

In 2007, the World Health Organization (WHO) reported a connection between statin use and ALS. In sorting through Vigibase, a WHO database that tracks reports of adverse reactions to drugs throughout the world, Edwards and his colleagues found 43 reports of the development of ALS or an ALS-like disorder in people taking a statin. The paper's publication led to a front-page story in the July 3 edition of the Wall Street Journal.

Statins, Neuromuscular Degenerative Disease and an Amyotrophic Lateral Sclerosis-Like Syndrome

An Analysis of Individual Case Safety Reports from Vigibase

I. Ralph Edwards, Kristina Star and *Anne Kiuru*

The WHO Foundation Collaborating Centre for International Drug Monitoring, the Uppsala Monitoring Centre (UMC), Uppsala, Sweden

Results: 'Upper motor neurone lesion' is a rare adverse event reported in relationship to drugs in Vigibase (a database containing nearly 4 million ICSRs). Of the total of 172 ICSRs on this reported term, 43 were related to statins, of which 40 were considered further: all but one case was reported as ALS. In 34/40 reports a statin was the sole reported suspected drug. The diagnostic criteria were variable, and seven of the statin cases also had features of peripheral neuropathy.

Drug Safety 2007; 30 (6): 515-525
0114-5916/07/0006-0515/$44.95/0

Similar results are found in the FDA's Adverse Events Reports (AERs). Of 10,086 AERs attributed to only one statin (Merck's

Zocor) over 13 years, 4,241 cases (24%) were nerve and brain related.

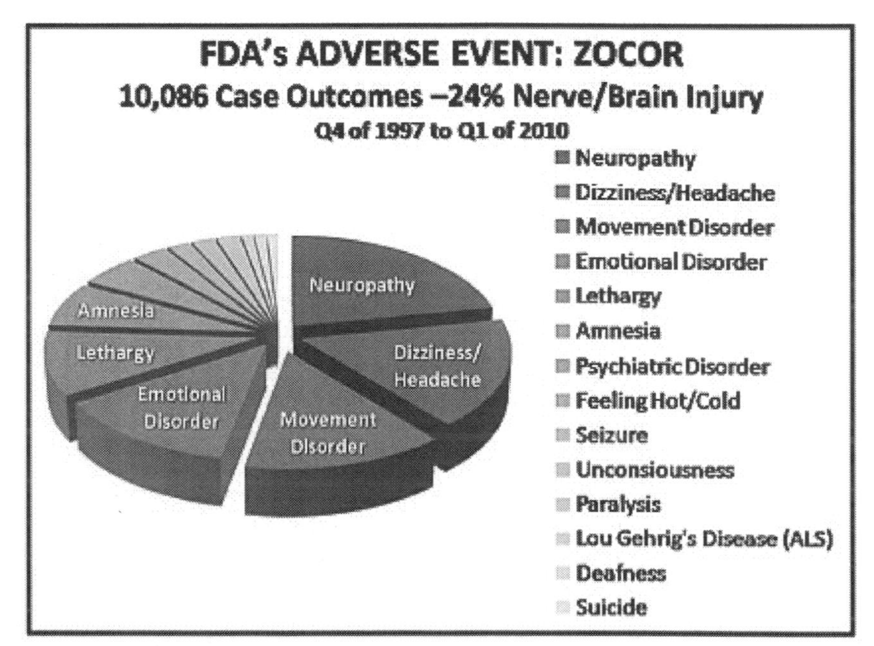

Of those 4,241 nerve/brain related statin-induced injuries, 59 had been diagnosed as Zocor-induced ALS (this represents reporting for only *one* statin brand of many):

Summary of Reaction Preferred Terms	# of Cases
LETHARGY	466
DIZZINESS/HEADACHE	703
NEUROPATHY	943
MEMORY/COGNITIVE LOSS	298
MOVEMENT DISORDER	612
EMOTION CHANGE	539
FEELING HOT/COLD	147
SEIZURE	86
UNCONSCIOUSNESS	67
PSYCHIATRIC SYMPTOM	193
PARALYSIS	87
LOU GEHRIG'S DISEASE (ALS)	**59**
DEAFNESS	24
SUICIDE	17

Because the connection between mycotoxin (statin) and ALS is rarely made, ***these numbers are grossly underreported.***

In 2010, PBS aired *The Suicide Tourist*, which chronicled Mary and Craig Colby Ewert's trip to Switzerland where assisted suicide is yet legal. Ewert's story of his battle with ALS was heart rending. Up until the day he decidedly chose to die, the camera recorded him compliantly ingesting his daily medication; I couldn't help but wonder if he had been prescribed a statin.

While many mycotoxins lower blood cholesterol, they also increase cholesterol inside cells with LDL cholesterol receptors (reference 37). Statins, in particular, work to lower blood cholesterol by moving cholesterol from the blood into cells of the liver and other tissue beds such as the muscles. Elevated cholesterol in cells is toxic and can cause apoptosis or programmed cell death. When this happens in muscle cells (as seen with metastatic cancer and statin myopathy) it causes muscle wasting. Statin-injured muscle has been described as "mush" (reference 38).

Effects of lipoprotein lipase and statins on cholesterol uptake into heart and skeletal muscle

Masayoshi Yokoyama,* Toru Seo,† Taesik Park,* Hiroaki Yagyu,* Yunying Hu,* Ni Huiping Son,* Ayanna S. Augustus,* Reeba K. Vikramadithyan,* Rajasekhar Ramakrishnan,† Leslie K. Pulawa,§ Robert H. Eckel,§ and Ira J. Goldberg[1,*]

In mice with greater LDL uptake resulting from muscle overexpression of LPL, statin therapy increased LDL uptake and tissue cholesterol content and caused muscle damage. Increased cellular cholesterol can lead to dysfunction or even apoptosis (8).

March 2007 The Journal of Lipid Research, 48, 646-655.

Apoptosis of muscle cells by mycotoxins provides a definitive mechanism for muscle atrophy (amyotropy) in statin-induced and similar mycotoxin induced cases of ALS. ***Amyotrophy and motor neuron degeneration in statin users is proof for this connection***. Apoptosis of motor nerve cells by apoptosis likewise provides an explanation for motor nerve destruction in mycotoxin-induced ALS.

Statin-Associated Myopathy with Normal Creatine Kinase Levels

Paul S. Phillips, MD; Richard H. Haas, MD; Sergei Bannykh, MD, PhD; Stephanie Hathaway, RN; Nancy L. Gray, RN; Bruce J. Kimura, MD; Georgirene D. Vladutiu, PhD; John D.F. England, MD; and the Scripps Mercy Clinical Research Center*

A muscle biopsy performed during atorvastatin therapy revealed increased lipid droplets, ragged red fibers, and cytochrome oxidase-negative muscle fibers, all consistent with lipid myopathy.

Ann Intern Med 2002;136:501-505

In fact, the Japanese developer of the first statin reported that in 1977 (the era of the mycotoxin gold rush when drug companies were scrambling to find ways to market mycotoxins) statin development almost stopped after cholesterol crystals were found accumulating and crystallizing inside cells of experimental animals. The find was eventually dismissed as "nontoxic cholesterol crystals" and work resumed. Three years later cancer reportedly developed in half their lab dogs (yes, mycotoxins cause cancer too). Work stopped. But the father of statins, Akira Endo, was a driven man. He pressed on with clandestine human trials and then published "positive" cholesterol lowering results; mycotoxin gold fever set in and statin development resumed.

A gift from nature: the birth of the statins

Akira Endo

We encountered a second challenge in April 1977. The issue was the detection of microcrystalline structures in the liver cells of rats that had been fed extremely large amounts of compactin (more than 500 milligrams per kilogram body weight per day (mg/kg/d)) for 5 weeks. The toxicologists insisted that these structures were toxic substances. It took us 9 months to identify these microcrystalline structures as nontoxic cholesterol.

There is no such thing as "nontoxic cholesterol *crystals*" accumulating inside cells. Furthermore, it is a bad idea to ingest a pathogenic mycotoxin to lower one's blood cholesterol. To further understand the mechanism of how statins destroy cells and cause amyotrophy, read: "How Statin Drugs Really Lower Cholesterol *And Kill You One Cell at a Time*".

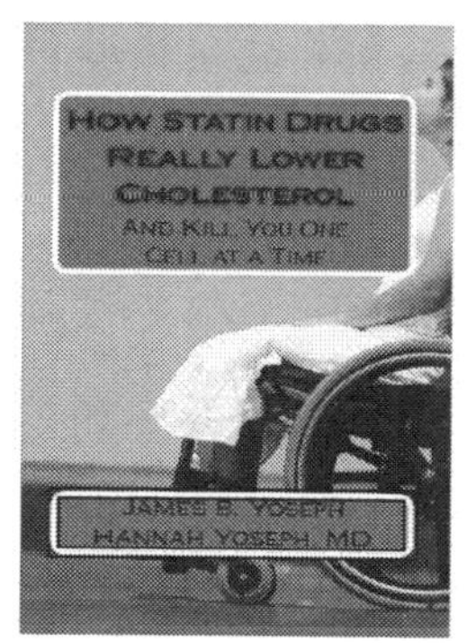

Mankind's mycotoxin madness has expanded to marketing them as "fungal biological control agents" – or FBCA. They are used as herbicides in foreign lands to defoliate opium poppies and as pesticides for farm crops. We spray mycotoxins everywhere – and have been doing it for decades. Even genetically modified versions of Aspergillus flavus toxins are sold for gain. FBCA are sold as "all-natural" insecticides. We buy them and spray them on our crops and coat our oranges with them to extend shelf life. They are indiscriminately applied as weed killers to ball fields without giving second thought to the athletes who then roll in it.

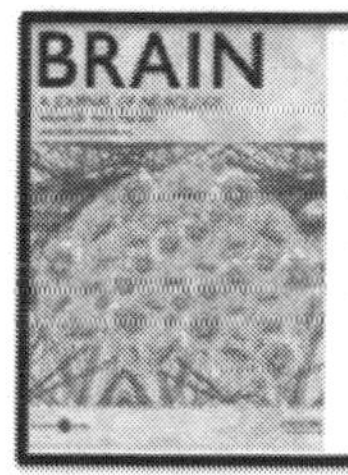

Severely Increased Risk of Amyotrophic Lateral Sclerosis Among Italian Professional Football Players.

Brain, 2005: 128 (3): 472-76.

Predictably, multiple studies demonstrate a relationship between exposure to agricultural chemicals and ALS.

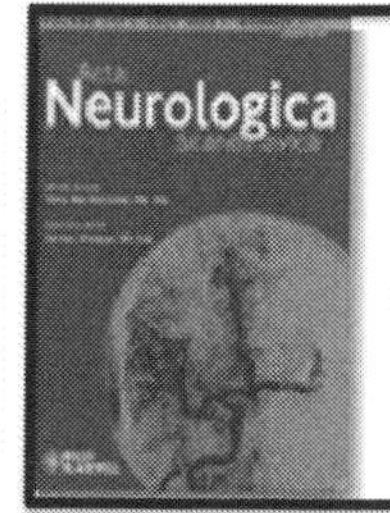

Amyotrophic Lateral Sclerosis in Sweden in Relation to Occupation

Gunnarsson L, Lindberg G, Soderfeldt B, Axelson O.

Acta Neurologica Scandinavica, 1991: 83 (6): 394-98.

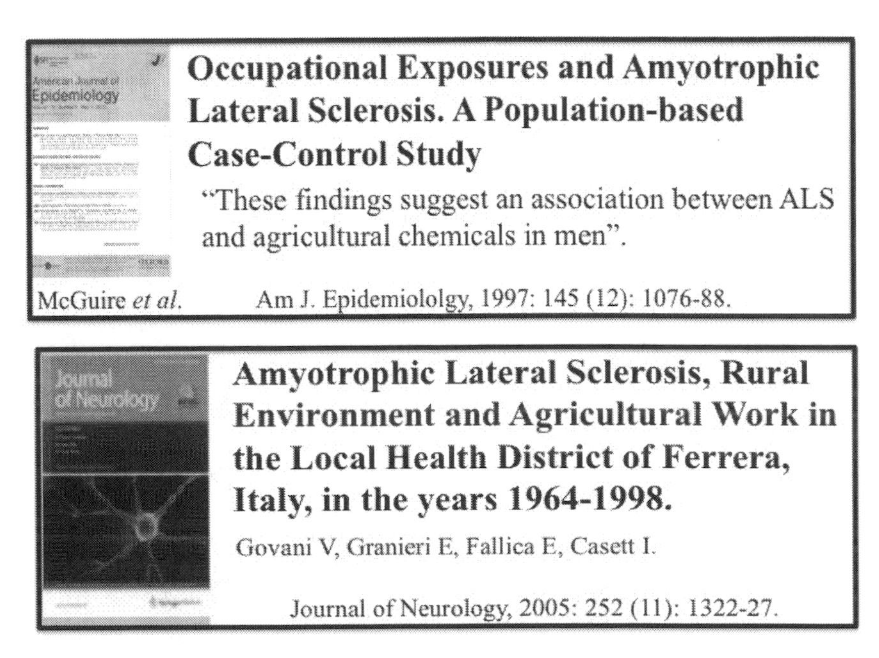
Occupational Exposures and Amyotrophic Lateral Sclerosis. A Population-based Case-Control Study

"These findings suggest an association between ALS and agricultural chemicals in men".

McGuire *et al.* Am J. Epidemiololgy, 1997: 145 (12): 1076-88.

Amyotrophic Lateral Sclerosis, Rural Environment and Agricultural Work in the Local Health District of Ferrera, Italy, in the years 1964-1998.

Govani V, Granieri E, Fallica E, Casett I.

Journal of Neurology, 2005: 252 (11): 1322-27.

Bad news: mycotoxins cause ALS. Good news: some mycotoxicity is reversible. Also, as a result of widespread statin use, a whole host of autoimmune and other degenerative diseases can now be *clearly* attributed to mycotoxin toxicity.

Statins, like other like-acting and reversible mycotoxins, also block cells from making CoQ10 which is essential to the energy cycle. Instead of being burned in the energy cycle, dietary acid wastes increase in cells; this provides an environment that promotes mycotoxin accumulation, opportunistic infection proliferation and degenerative disease progression. This will be further explained in Part Three after First Steps to follow.

Bottom line: The evidence of mycotoxins' causal relationship to ALS is clear. There are many mycotoxins that cause ALS like symptoms. More work needs to be done to discover antidotes to mycotoxins such as territrem-B that irreversibly bind to acetylcholinesterase. For cases of ALS such as statin-induced ALS where mycotoxin action on cells is reversible, there is hope for remedy. It is time, now, to take off blinders and find cure(s).

Chapter 13: First Steps

"Patience is a virtue wasted on the old and fishermen."
-Don Wright

Cleaning up your swimming pool so that it is no longer friendly to disease-causing CWD bacteria and mycotoxins is not about will power. It is about knowing a little about basic chemistry and being patient.

Basically, you want your body water (water inside cells, tissue and blood) to be basic. The only test you need to determine progress is how you feel.

As your water is slowly corrected to a basic pH of an average 7.4, the tiny oxygen-hating microbes will die. This will both release toxins and activate the immune system to clean up the debris (dead microbes and damaged tissue). This, at first, may make you feel worse than better. The symptoms of an alarmed immune system are similar to a cold or chronic infection: fatigue, fever, headaches, muscle aches, etc.

If these symptoms are too uncomfortable, simply stop or taper back on these first steps to follow. If you are still taking drugs that suppress the immune system, the symptoms of an activated immune system may be further aggravated. The choice is ultimately yours. It is, after all, your life! Either way, good PH levels and good nutrition is do no harm medicine.

One of the most powerful and overlooked antibiotics are alkaline minerals which "buffer" water so that pH remains basic. Use nature's antibiotic to nurture your cells back to health. This chapter includes the "first steps" for slowly making your body water basic. This should be done before adding the "second steps" of chapter 29. Patience is key.

The following protocol is for a minimum of two weeks – before starting the second steps in chapter 29. First steps are about changing body water with fluids; second steps are about changing body water with food and food supplements.

FIRST STEPS

1. Avoid all oxidizers such as chlorine, fluoride and phosphoric acid that destroy life-essential isoprenoids such as cell membranes. This means NO city tap water (well water is okay) and NO soft drinks (soda pop).

2. Avoid all acidic drinks. This means NO soft drinks (diet or regular), no black coffee and no black tea. If you have problems with caffeine-withdrawal headaches, add plenty of milk or cream to your coffee or tea to raise the pH. Try to taper back and preferably even quit until you are feeling better. ***NEVER ingest soft drinks or tap water for the rest of your life no matter how good you feel.*** If you want to kill some marine life, put them in a tank of chlorinated water (or soda) – and watch them die.

3. Avoid all bottled drinks/juices, sports drinks, powdered drink mixes and distilled water.

4. Drink lots of clean well water or bottled spring water. Do not drink bottled water that has been purified by "reverse osmosis" or "distillation". These so-called "purification" techniques remove alkaline mineral such as calcium and magnesium from water. Of all the bottled waters that I've tested, Evian is the most mineral rich (and readily found).

5. Drink lots of freshly-made fruit juice, made mostly with apples (more about this in Part Two).

6. Alka-Seltzer or no-brand substitute (plain or lemon flavored): one packet (two tablets) in water as directed two to four times daily until feeling better.

7. If you used to be addicted to soft drinks, seltzer water is a safe substitute. This can be flavored with fresh-squeezed lemon or lime and sweetened with stevia (if needed).

8. 1,000 mg of calcium citrate capsules or as directed: take at night with food (these can cause fatigue).

9. 500 mg of magnesium malate capsules or as directed: take in morning with food (these can energize).

10. Use salt which contains sodium – another alkaline mineral. (Exception: If you have problems with edema such as ankle swelling, then avoid salt until this is resolved.)

To sum, during the health restoration process, do the following:

DRINK:

Spring or well water
Fresh-squeezed apple juice
Seltzer water
Green, herbal and fruit teas (with or without caffeine)

SUPPLEMENT WITH ALKALINE (BASIC) MINERALS:

Calcium citrate capsules (night)
Magnesium malate capsules (morning)
Salt on food
Alka-Seltzer (at least twice daily)
Cell Food (add to drinks as directed)

Remember, don't try to monitor your progress by using pH strips to test saliva or urine pH. These tests do not accurately reflect the pH of tissue water. Dietary acids are filtered through the kidneys into the urine, so an acidic urine pH does not reflect the pH of tissue beds (such as muscle). Saliva pH is altered by the pH of food or drink. ***The best test is how you feel.***

These first steps focus on how *fluids* affect your body water. Part Two explains how *foods* affect your body water.

In Part One, you learned that less hydrogen in water leaves more oxygen in water to evict disease causing CWD microbes that hate oxygen. In Part Two, you will learn that it is the power of vitamins in carbohydrate foods that determines whether pure energy is made from carbs or just a little bit of energy and a lot of acid waste that further contaminates your body water (and feeds the "mosquitoes").

It is the power of hydrogen in carbohydrate foods, and how efficiently the hydrogen is metabolized, that either turns your water into an acid wasteland or energizes your life. This requires a solid understanding of how food is metabolized into energy (Part Two) – or acid. And you already know what likes acid; it isn't you!

Bottom Line: CWD bacteria, yeast and fungi hate alkaline-rich oxygenated basic water. Make your body water (swimming pool) an unfriendly environment for these toxin producing parasites. Remember, a basic pH is nature's antibiotic!

PART TWO: COSMICALLY-SIMPLE ENERGY

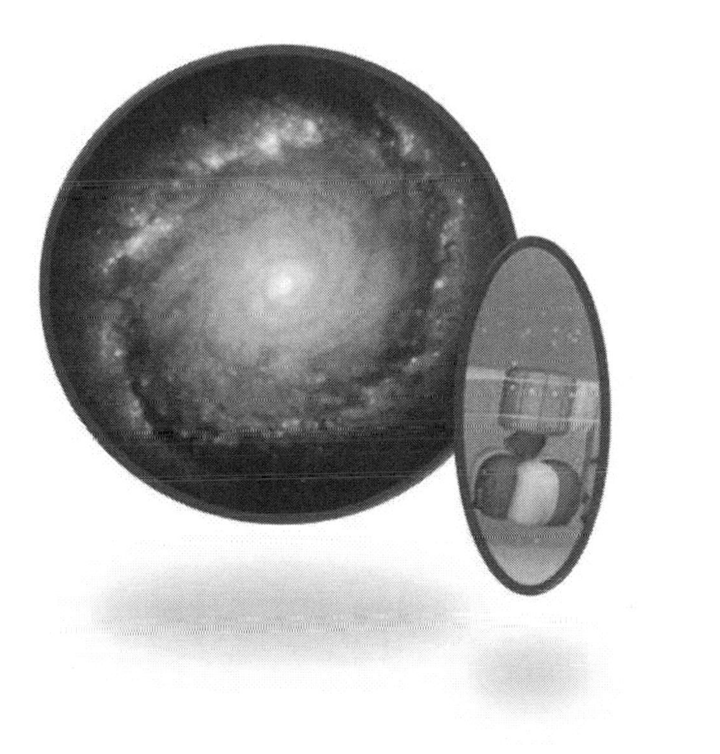

Chapter 14: Hydrogen Fuel

"To eat is a necessity, but to eat intelligently is an art."
-La Rochefoucauld

The food that you eat, just like the fluids that you drink, can either feed or starve the CWD bacteria implicated in autoimmune syndromes. What all of these tiny microbes share in common is that they thrive in acidic poorly-oxygenated water.

Food, like fluids that you drink, can make your body water acidic and feed the bugs or can make your body water basic and starve them. To understand how food affects the pH of your body water requires a few lessons about an important molecule called "ATP".

Carbohydrates convert into the energy molecule abbreviated as ATP. When you understand how cells make it, you will see how ATP is the ultimate source of "**A**ll **T**rue **P**ower" for healthy cells.

Every cell in your body needs ATP to perform its particular function – be it a heart cell to pump your blood, a nerve cell to keep you awake or a muscle cell to move your body. When your cells make enough ATP, they have the energy needed to function normally – and that makes for a healthy you!

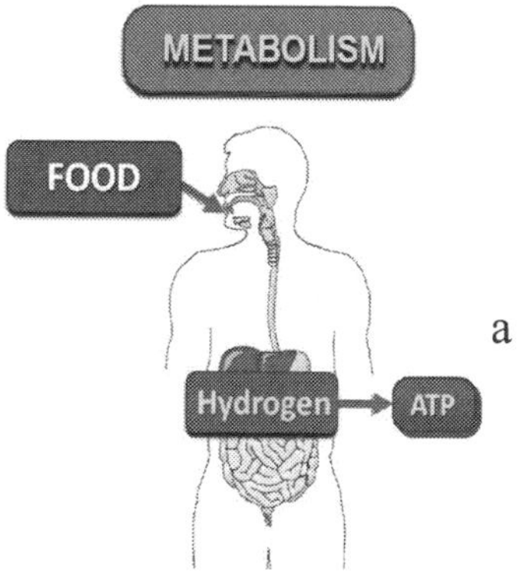

Cells manufacture ATP from hydrogen from the food you eat. The process of making ATP from hydrogen is called *metabolism*.

Optimum ATP production is the key to a healthy metabolism and a lean and healthy body. That is because food that is not metabolized into ATP instead makes dietary acids instead of energy.

ATP, the body's energy molecule, works like a rechargeable battery that makes energy for every cell. When cells generate ATP efficiently, you will be lean and full of energy rather than sick and tired and stuffing up some doctor's office waiting to get a bunch of prescription pills that will never clean your swimming pool and promote a healthy metabolism.

ATP is the fuel you need to move, eat, think and sleep. Without sufficient ATP, you simply cannot be healthy. And, more likely than not, you will also be overweight, sore, tired and frequently sick.

Optimum ATP production is the key to overall health – period!

ATP production, or cellular metabolism, is made primarily from carbohydrate foods that are broken down into carbon dioxide and hydrogen. The ***carbo*** portion of ***carbo***hydrates makes ***carbon dioxide***, which is exhaled. The ***hydrate*** portion of carbo***hydrates*** releases ***hydrogen*** that is converted into ATP.

Humans are energized by hydrogen from food that makes ATP.

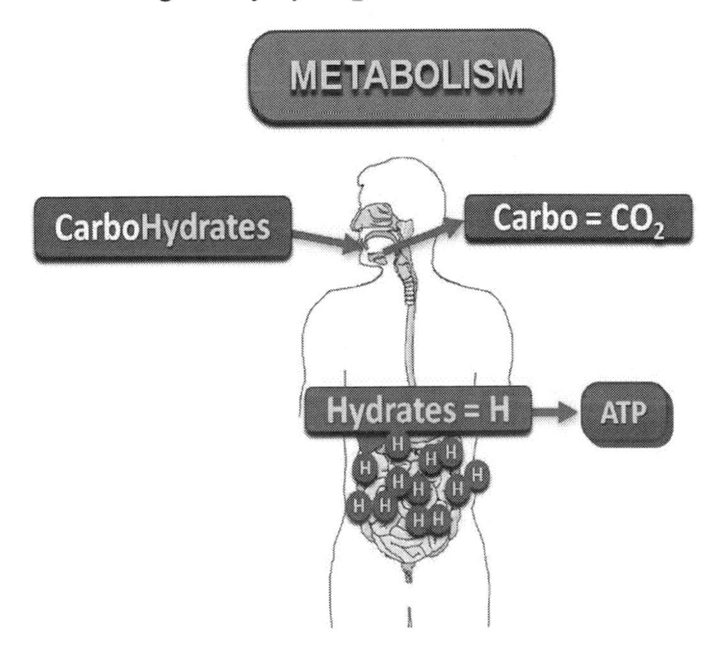

ATP can be made in cells without oxygen (anaerobic metabolism or *glycolysis*) or with oxygen (aerobic metabolism or *oxidation*). Oxidation makes 18 times more ATP than glycolysis.

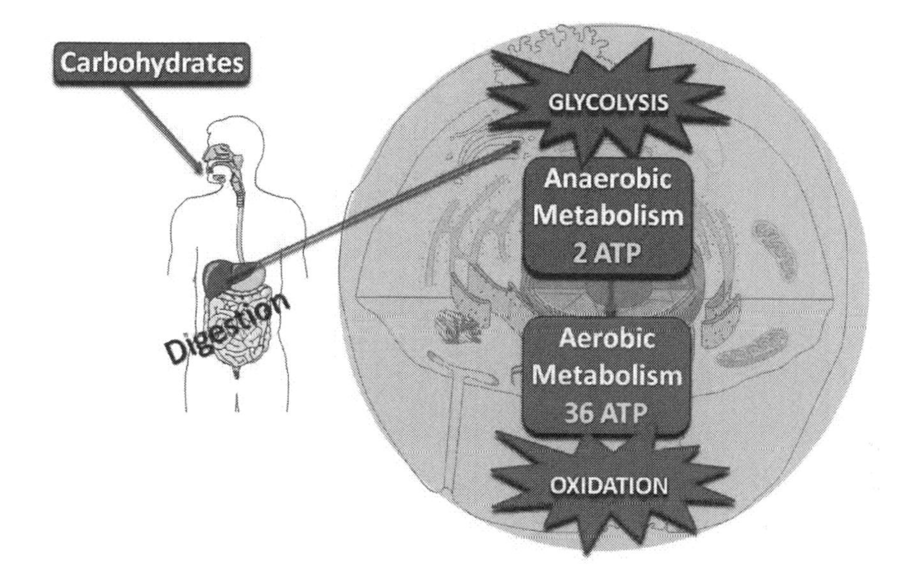

Did you catch that? ***Oxidation makes 18 times more ATP than glycolysis!*** If you're overweight, frequently sick, fatigued and suffer from stiff and sore muscles, then your cells are likely stuck in the energy-deficient and fat-making mode of glycolysis rather than the energy-making and health-promoting mode of oxidation.

Notably, CWD microbes prefer to make ATP by glycolysis which further compromises cellular health.

Bottom Line: Metabolism (glycolysis and oxidation) is the process of converting food into ATP to make cellular energy. ATP is the energy molecule that every cell in your body needs to function normally.

Chapter 15: Energy for Life

"Energy is eternal delight."
-William Blake

Most all the energy to operate your bio-computer (brain) comes from glucose. Glucose is a carbohydrate. Lack of glucose activates the hunger reflex. That is why "low carb" diets don't work. Eventually you surrender to the hunger reflex. And you should. It is essential to life.

Low carb diets are like trying to hold your breath. You will either voluntarily submit to the reflexive drive to breathe, or pass out and breathe involuntarily. Either way, you will breathe again!

The body makes energy from carbohydrates. If not enough nutritional carbohydrates are consumed, cells will convert fat and protein to carbohydrates (glucose). That is another reason why low carb diets do not work. Without consuming enough nutritious carbohydrates, the hunger reflex is never completely satisfied. A full belly will not turn off the food craving. The brain continually nags with hunger. It is designed to do so.

Hydrogen, from carbo***hydrates*** (foods made of carbon and hydrogen) makes ATP for every cell in your body. ***Hydrogen, the energy source of ATP, is what primarily determines whether you are healthy or sick, lean or fat and energized or fatigued.***

In fact, hydrogen not only energizes you…it energizes the universe!

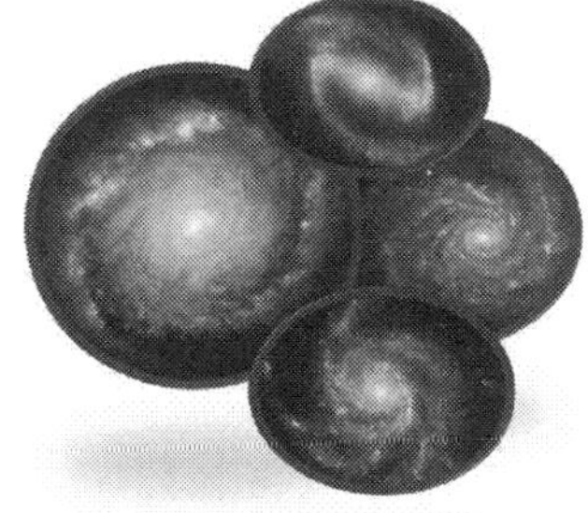

Energy from hydrogen is what lights up the stars – and lights up your life. From atoms to galaxies to making energy in your cells, hydrogen, the tiniest atom on planet earth, is spinning and energizing everything.

Every cell in your body is a microscopic universe of spinning hydrogen atoms making billions of ATP molecules every minute. Each cell contains tens to thousands of ATP factories that look like peanut-shaped swimming pools called mitochondria (pronounced *mite-o-kon-dree-ah*). The number of these depends on the energy needs of a cell. A skin cell, for example, has tens of mitochondria whereas a heart cell can have thousands of them. It is inside these peanut-shaped pools of water-like matrix that ATP, the energy molecule of life, is made from hydrogen from the food you eat.

Mitochondria look like pools with a double-liner – with inner and outer membranes. These peanut-shaped pools are batteries that accumulate hydrogen in the space between the membranes. As hydrogen builds up under "pressure", it flows into the matrix – and it is this movement of hydrogen that makes ATP.

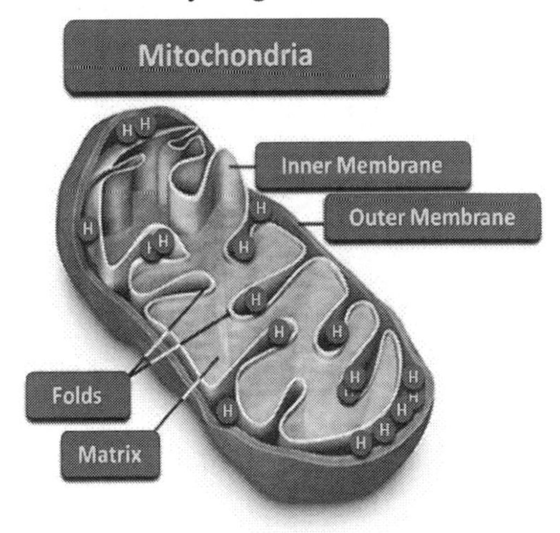

This process is similar to how water is used to make electricity. In a hydroelectric dam, flowing water spins turbines that generate electricity. In mitochondria, dammed-up hydrogen atoms flow to turn turbine-like molecules that spin to make ATP.

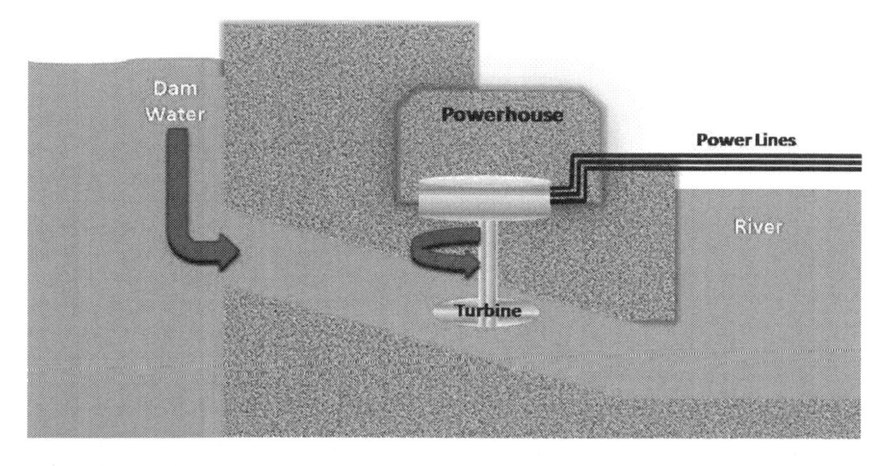

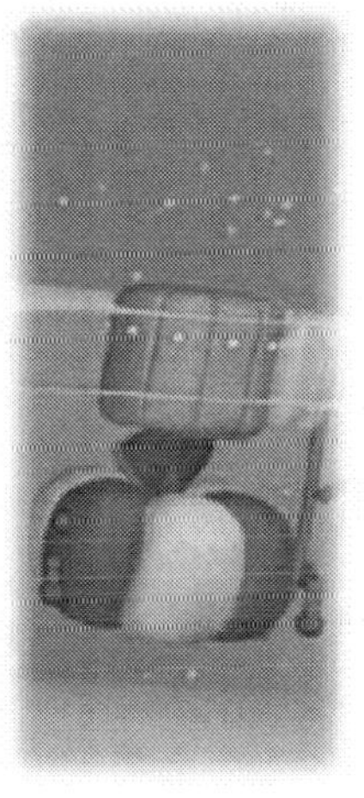

The spinning turbine-like molecules that synthesize ATP are called *ATP Synthase*. ATP Synthase is one of the most amazing molecules because it literally *spins* as hydrogen flows through it. The energy from this spinning action is what makes ATP – the energy molecule of life.

Living things store energy mainly in the form of chemical bonds. ATP contains a high-energy chemical bond that is used by all cells to do work. When energy is released from ATP, it converts to ADP – which is the "uncharged" form of ATP. Every minute, every cell converts billions of ATP molecules into ADP plus energy. ATP Synthase then converts ADP back into ATP – like a rechargeable battery – so that the process can continue over and over again.

Carbohydrates are the main source of hydrogen for making ATP. Interestingly, not all carbohydrates are created equal in regards to their ATP-making potential. This is where money matters. Cheap (inexpensive) processed carbohydrates that are stripped of the nutrients needed to completely metabolize into ATP, will make acids instead of hydrogen – and it is those incompletely metabolized acids that feed acid-loving microbes. These acids can also be converted into fat (from fatty acids).

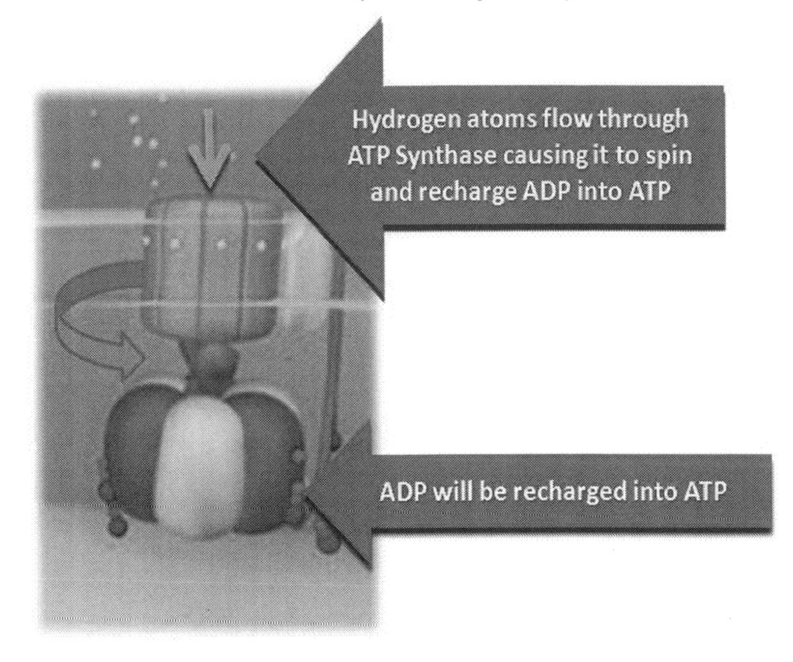

It is the highly-nutritious, unprocessed carbohydrates that one can eat without counting calories. These foods make plenty of ATP and maintain the oxygen-rich basic water pH that chokes the life out of Chlamydia pneumoniae.

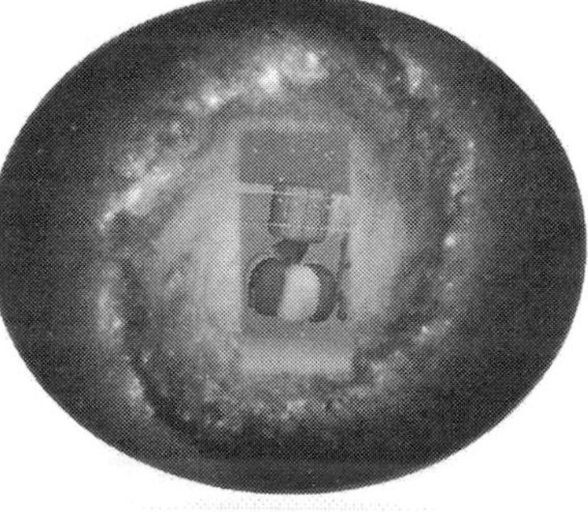

Bottom Line: Every cell is a universe of mobile hydrogen atoms that spin ATP Synthase to make ATP – the energy molecule of life. ***Hydrogen comes from carbohydrates which do not make ATP equally; in fact, some can only make acids which, in turn, feed oxygen-hating acid-loving CWD bacteria – that produce more acids.***

Chapter 16: An Apple a Day

"He who has health has hope which is everything."
-Ancient Proverb

From spiral galaxies to mitochondria, hydrogen is spinning and energizing the universe. When the spinning slows down, you can lose your nerve. When acid instead of ATP is made, CWD bacteria can proliferate. These don't have any nerve, but to live they need the "stuff" that your nerves are made of.

The ALS diet is not about counting calories; it is about eating foods that make the maximum amount of energy. Certain carbohydrates, such as the ordinary apple and onion, are so nutrient-rich that they always metabolize into maximum ATP instead of fat and dietary acid wastes. Stiff, sore, tired or gaining weight? Eat some raw apples or top raw diced onion on your cooked food! It's no coincidence that for hundreds of years, folks observed that "an apple a day keeps the doctor away" – but eat as many as you want!

Armed with a practical knowledge of how carbohydrates convert into hydrogen, when you reach for foods like the amazing apple and onion that are so packed with ATP-making power, that the more you eat the more energy you will have, the more fat you will lose (if overweight) and the more health you will enjoy.

Carbohydrates or "carbs" (fruits, vegetables and grains) are the chemical energy source of all cells. All carbohydrates are digested, absorbed into the blood and then routed to the liver where they are packaged into a simple sugar called *glucose.* An apple, carrot and bagel, then, all end up in the blood as glucose. ***Glucose is your fuel...but if and only IF it is thoroughly metabolized into hydrogen to make energy as ATP.***

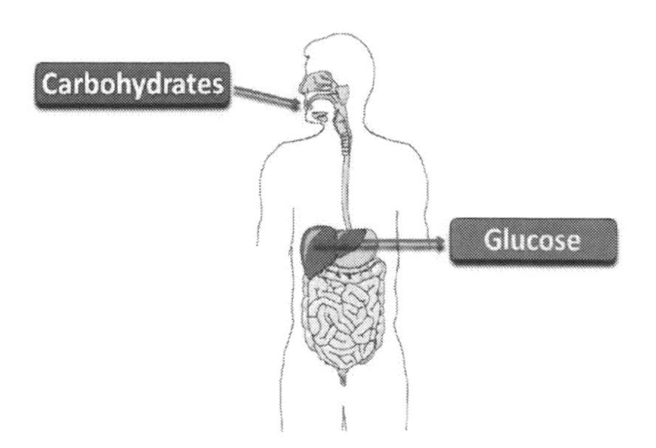

From the liver, glucose circulates in the blood to cells of organs and tissues where it is split into acids. The process of splitting glucose in half is called *glycolysis* (*lysis* means *to split*) and the acid product is *pyruvic acid*. Just like the splitting of logs releases energy to warm an ax-head, the splitting of glucose releases energy to make a small amount of ATP – 2 units for every unit of glucose. ***Pyruvic acid can be further oxidized to make 36 more units of ATP – but only if there is sufficient oxygen and nutrients in the cell...and that's a big IF!***

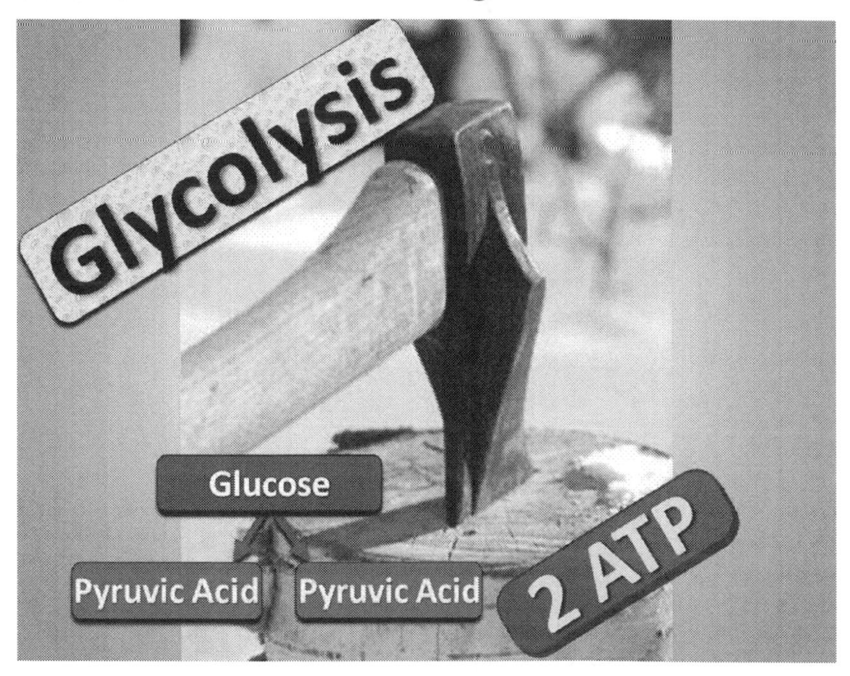

Wood is a carbohydrate. A log of wood burns (oxidizes) more efficiently if first split. Glycolysis, then, is like wood-splitting; this takes place in cell water where miniscule amounts of ATP are made by the energy that is released when glucose is split into smaller molecules of acid.

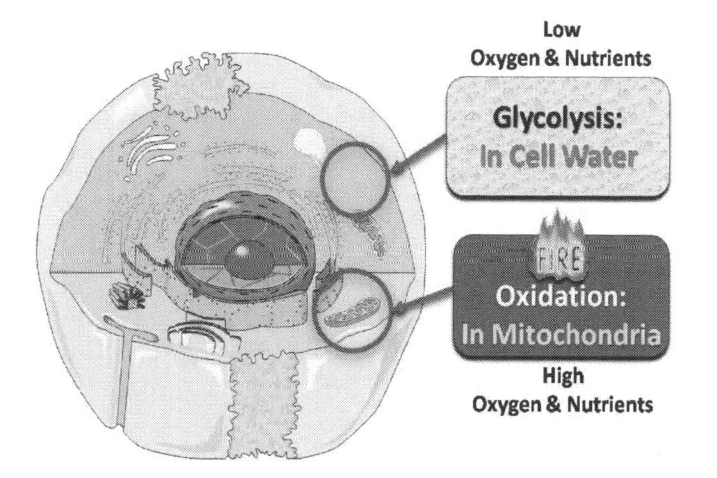

Oxidation, on the other hand, takes place in mitochondria, and this is where the real "fire" of metabolism takes place.

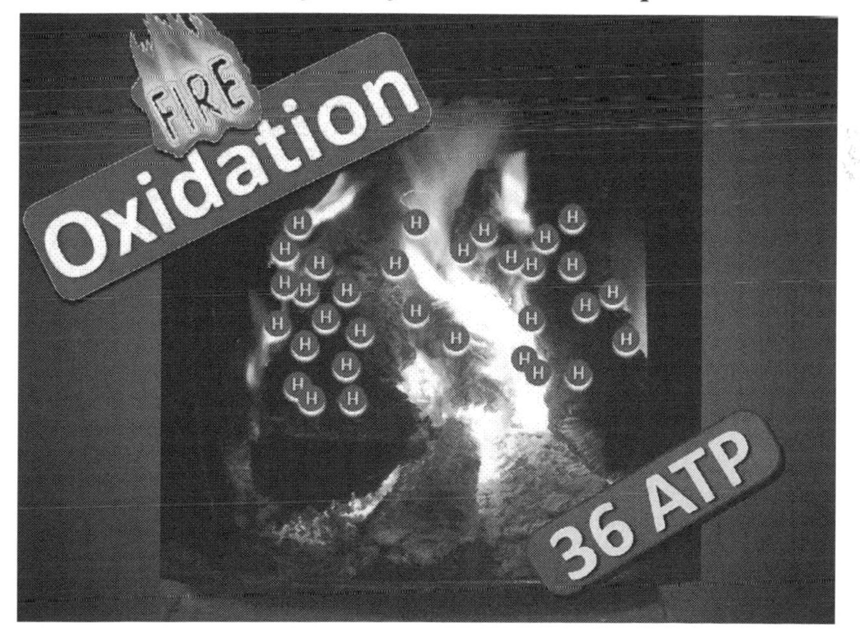

Chlamydia pneumoniae swim inside the cell water (not the mitochondria where oxidation occurs) and make energy primarily by glycolysis; they are acid-making factories.

Since much more ATP is made by oxidation within mitochondria, the key to cellular health (and losing excess fat which is an acid) is found in charging up your mitochondria with nutrients and oxygen. This will ensure that carbohydrates make only hydrogen and ATP instead of acid wastes.

Glycolysis does not require oxygen or many nutrients.

Oxidation, on the other hand, requires oxygen and *many* nutrients, just like a fire requires oxygen and properly-seasoned wood to burn well.

Nutrient-rich carbohydrates that completely oxidize make 18 times more ATP than by glycolysis!

Bottom Line: All carbohydrates are converted in the liver into a simple sugar called glucose which is then split into acids inside the water of cells by glycolysis. If sufficient nutrients and oxygen are present within cells, the acid products of glycolysis will oxidize to make 18 times more energy as ATP.

Fat and degenerative illness is a four-letter word: ACID.

Chapter 17: Keep the Cycle Burning

"Health and cheerfulness naturally beget each other."
-Joseph Addison

If CWD bacteria are like mosquitoes in a stagnant pool, then clean water and nutrients will flush them out.

Oxygen and nutrients are required to completely oxidize glucose into energy rather than dietary acids and fat. If you are tired, sore, weak and/or overweight, what is lacking are nutrients and oxygen-rich basic water that fuels a healthy metabolism.

After glucose is split (glycolysis), pyruvic acid enters the mitochondria and is further degraded to the smaller molecule *Acetyl-CoA* (*ah-see-till-co-ay*). Acetyl-CoA represents a major crossroad for all carbohydrate consumers as this molecule is the building block for making energy as ATP – or making dietary acids wastes. The path taken by acetyl-CoA depends on what nutrients are available in the food that was eaten.

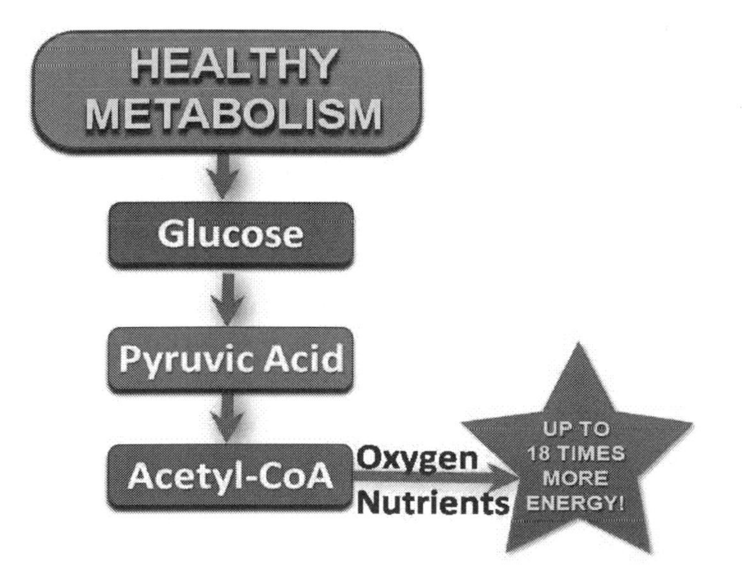

Depending on the nutrients in the ingested carbohydrate, acetyl-CoA can turn into energy (ATP) or anergy (acid).

A healthy metabolism, based upon eating as much as you want of carefully selected foods, will always make more energy whether you exercise or not! Aerobic exercising, which delivers more oxygen to cells, enhances oxidation just as do certain nutrients. Exercise does not guarantee a healthy metabolism; in fact, in cases of ALS and other autoimmune conditions where acid-making microbes are infecting cells, exercise will risk making more acids that exacerbate the infection (more on this later). ***If acetyl-CoA is blocked from oxidation for any reason, health is compromised because acid instead of ATP is made.***

For acetyl-CoA to stay in the mitochondria and make energy (rather than exit into the cell water and make fat), it combines with another dietary acid to make *citric acid* – the same acid that is found in citrus fruit. Citric acid is then oxidized (hydrogen atoms removed) until *malic acid* is formed – the same acid that is found in apples. Malic acid is then further oxidized until it recombines with acetyl-CoA again to make citric acid – and the cycle repeats again and again and again – ***if you eat enough nutritious food, that is, to keep this cycle burning.***

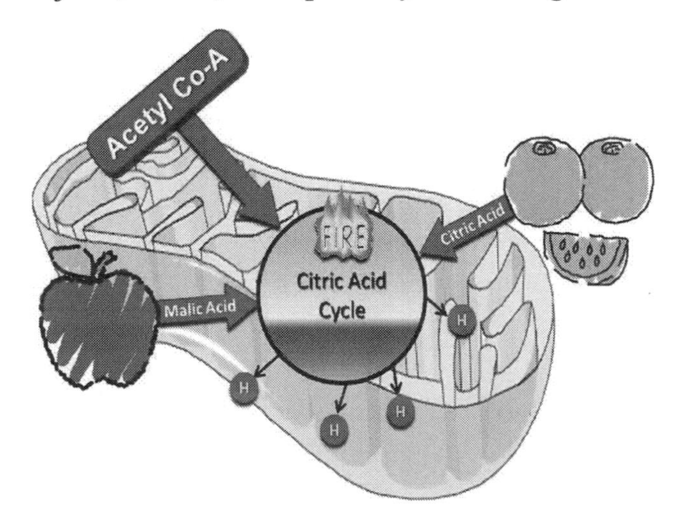

The conversion of citric acid to malic acid and back to citric acid is called the *citric acid cycle.* The oxidation of citric acid to malic acid releases *hydrogen atoms*, which are transported to the mitochondrial hydrogen dam for making ATP.

Acetyl-CoA is made from *acetic acid* – which is *vinegar.* Now you know why apple-cider vinegar, which contains malic acid (from apples) and acetic acid, is highly touted as a health and energy tonic – something our great grandmothers already knew before the citric acid cycle was discovered!

Bottom Line: After glycolysis, pyruvic acid enters the mitochondria where it is converted to *acetyl-CoA*. Acetyl-CoA fuels the citric acid cycle where citric acid is oxidized to release hydrogen atoms, which are transported to the mitochondrial hydrogen dam to make ATP. ***Foods such as vinegar, apples and oranges serve to keep the citric acid cycle burning. They are energy-making super-fuels.***

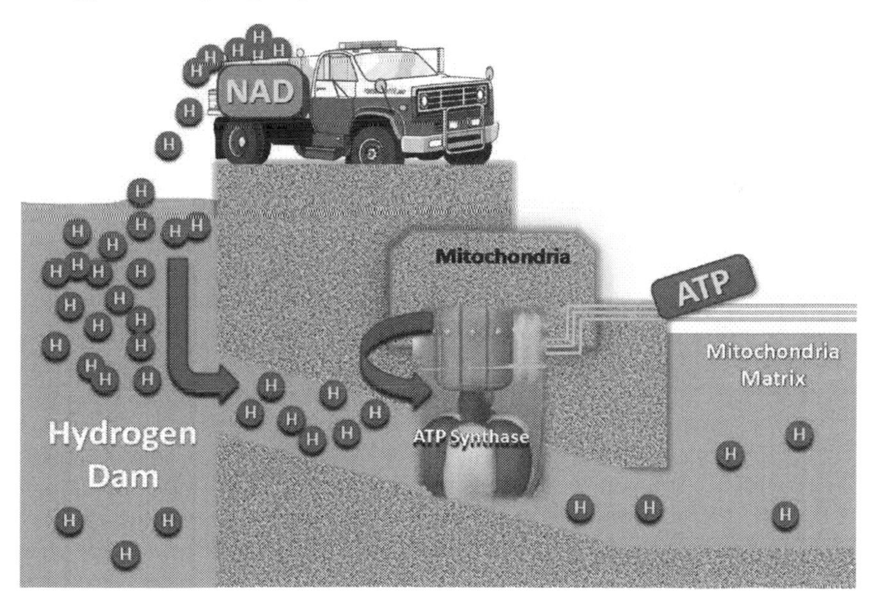

Chapter 18: The Beautiful B Vitamins

"True friendship is like sound health; the value of it is seldom known until lost."

-Charles Caleb Colton

As citric acid is oxidized to generate hydrogen atoms, hydrogen is delivered to the energy dam of the mitochondria (cell batteries) where it flows through ATP Synthase to make 95 percent of the potential ATP stored in glucose. The hydrogen atoms are transported to the dam by two molecules: FAD from vitamin B2 and NAD from vitamin B3.

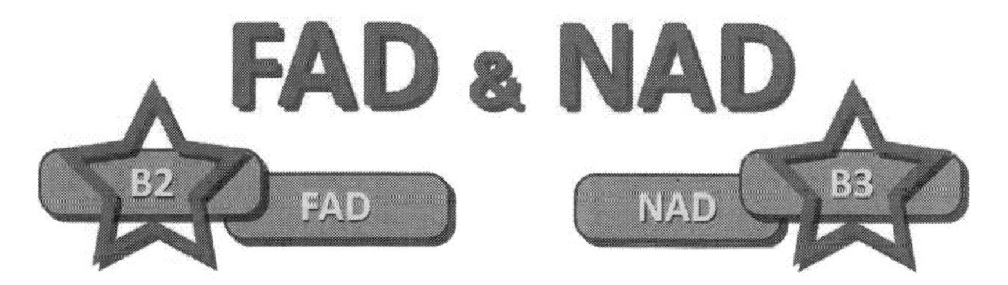

Vitamin B2 or ribo*F*lavin (the "F" in FAD) and vitamin B3 or *N*iacin (the "N" in NAD) are the carrier molecules that pick up hydrogen atoms from the citric acid cycle and deliver them to the hydrogen energy dam of the mitochondria.

Vitamins B2 and B3 are essential to making energy from carbs!

In a hydroelectric dam, stored-up water builds up pressure that is converted into power as electricity. In mitochondria, hydrogen is delivered (primarily by NAD) to the space between the double membranes of the mitochondria to build up hydrogen pressure that is converted into ATP. NAD is a much busier "cargo truck" than FAD as ninety percent of the hydrogen atoms are delivered by NAD.

Once hydrogen builds up sufficient pressure, it flows through ATP Synthase causing it to spin; this energy recharges ADP into ATP. ATP stands for Adenosine *Tri*-Phosphate (*Tri* meaning *Three*) and ADP is Adenosine *Di*-Phosphate (*Di* meaning *Two*). It is the *third* phosphate atom that gives ATP its energy "punch".

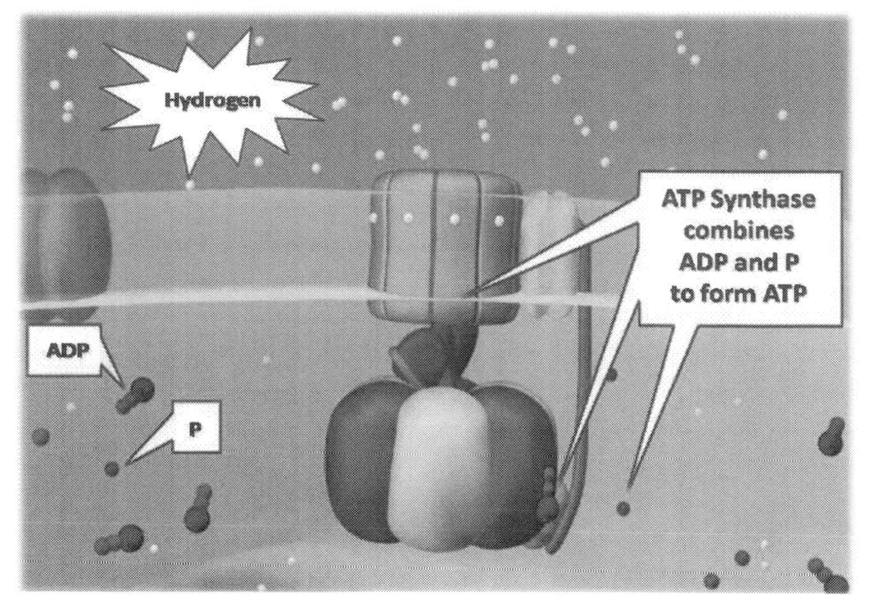

Foods rich in B2, B3 and phosphorus are all important sources, respectively, of FAD, NAD and ATP. When you do the math, vitamin B3 in the form of NAD is responsible for 80% of the ATP that cells can make (NAD delivers 90% of the hydrogen that is made into ATP in the mitochondria, but some ATP is also made by glycolysis; this accounts for the overall 80% contribution of vitamin B3 to ATP production).

Other B vitamins are also instrumental in metabolizing glucose. For example, the first step of glycolysis cannot occur without vitamin B1. Vitamin B5 makes up part of the molecule acetyl-CoA. FAD is made from vitamin B2. And most important of all is vitamin B3 to make NAD. Indeed, without an ample supply of the beautiful B vitamins floating around in cells, metabolism can be hindered or stopped at various stages, the result of which can even lead to death.

To be lean and healthy, the "fire" of the citric acid cycle needs to be well-fueled with NAD and other key nutrients. This ensures that carbohydrates are completely oxidized to make maximum hydrogen atoms to feed the ATP Synthase "batteries." Life or death, health or disease, is held closely in the balance in the mighty mitochondria.

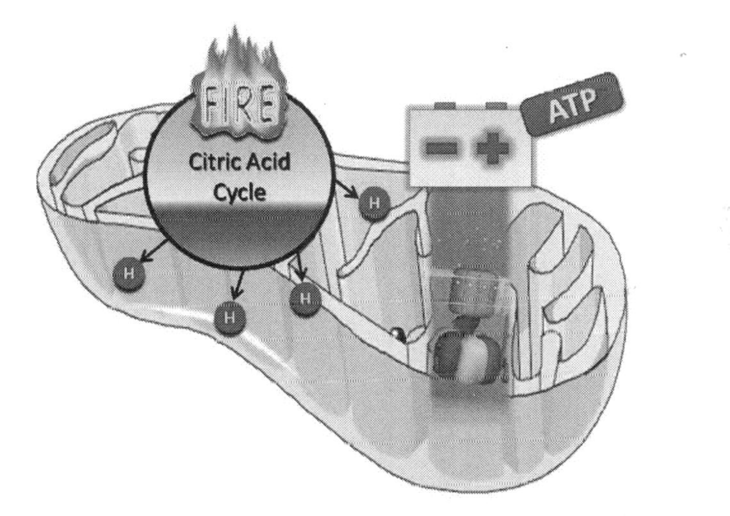

Bottom Line: Hydrogen atoms generated by the citric acid cycle are delivered to the mitochondrial hydrogen dam primarily by NAD which is derived from vitamin B3. ***NAD is responsible for 80% of the potential ATP that can be made from glucose.***

Chapter 19: Death by Deficiency

"Every day you do one of two things: build health or disease."
-Adelle Davis

In 1871, the city of Chicago nearly burned to the ground. A rumor circulated that Mrs. O'leary's cow kicked over an oil lamp, set her barn on fire and a strong night wind did the rest. Whether or not Mrs. O'leary's cow started the fire is not the issue. What is noteworthy is that Mrs. O'leary had a cow and a barn.

Up until the 1930's, it was common for people to have livestock, even in densely populated cities. Most people grew gardens in their back yards. Most all farms had an orchard. People followed their principle pursuit: food – albeit home grown and raised.

It was the pursuit of food that had spread humans all over the planet. By WWII, all of that began to radically change. In mass, women went to work in the defense and manufacturing industries. Home gardening became a thing of the past. Small farms began to disappear. Agriculture became big business. Canned, frozen and processed food met the need, and shelf life suddenly became critical. Foods shipped, warehoused and then stacked on shelves needed to not spoil – and active vitamins cause oxidation and spoilage. The predictable result was plagues of runaway obesity, cancer, heart disease, etc.

Back to the science of how *real* foods that quickly oxidize and therefore spoil can keep you energized, lean and healthy:

After glycolysis – the splitting of glucose – pyruvic acid enters the mitochondria where it is further degraded to the smaller molecule of acetyl-CoA. Acetyl-CoA enters the citric acid cycle where citric acid is oxidized (hydrogen atoms released) that are transported to the mitochondrial hydrogen dam. Ninety percent of the hydrogen atoms are transported by NAD to make 80% of the

ATP that can be made from a unit of glucose from carbohydrate food.

NAD – from vitamin B3 – is responsible for 80% of the potential ATP made from carbohydrates. Mitochondria are your batteries and ATP is your body's energy current. If your mitochondria aren't making enough ATP, you'll be like a low battery that can't start an engine.

While there are multiple nutritional deficiencies that can hinder ATP production, no single vitamin is as remarkable as B3 in terms of its overall contribution to ATP production – a whopping 80 percent.

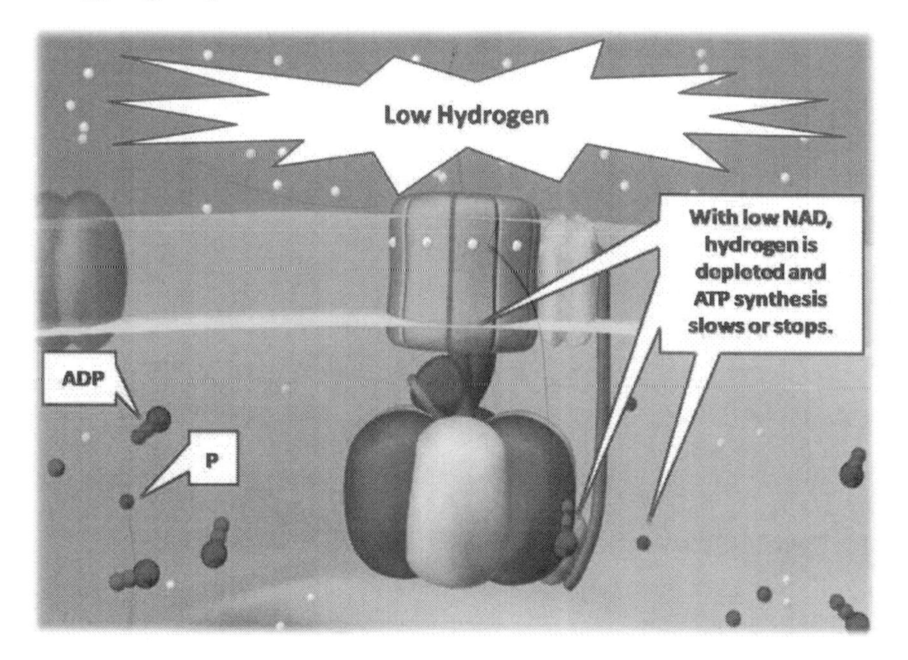

Without sufficient NAD to transport hydrogen to the energy-making dam, the hydrogen dam will be depleted and ATP production can come to a halt.

No ATP = no life.

If NAD deficiency becomes severe, organs will eventually fail to function as will the entire body. We call this *death.*

Considering the incalculable contribution that NAD makes to charge our cells' batteries, it is predictable that a severe deficiency in vitamin B3 can lead to death. The "four D's" of vitamin B3 deficiency (called "pellagra") are:

Diarrhea (irritable bowel)

Dermatitis (dry, scaly rash)

Dementia (mental fog and difficulty with thinking)

Death (but first comes chronic fatigue, sore muscles, problems with coordination...and *then* death).

With vitamin B3 as the main source of NAD, no wonder a deficiency in vitamin B3 can cause death. But before the fourth "**D**" of **D**eath tolls its bell, a whole host of other symptoms will surface as cell by cell and organ by organ, ATP production slows down.

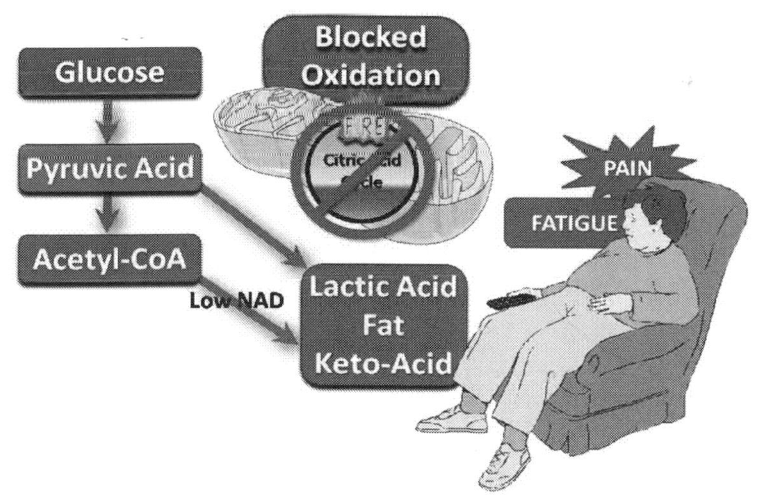

As long as a person breathes, in the face of an NAD deficiency ATP production can limp along by glycolysis alone – the product of which is a small amount of ATP and pyruvic acid which converts to other acids. ***One of these acids, called lactic acid, causes stiff and extremely tender muscles.*** Other acids such as keto-acids can cause coma and ultimately death. To further compound the problem, CWD bacteria thrive in an acidic environment. These make energy by glycolysis which further contributes to the acid wasteland. Good for them; bad for you.

The first "**D**" of vitamin B3 deficiency – **D**iarrhea – is usually the first symptom of NAD deficiency because the digestive system, which has a high demand for ATP for digesting and transporting food into the blood, is the first system to suffer ATP deficiency. Of all the organs of the digestive system, the pancreas has a very high demand for ATP to make enzymes for digesting and neutralizing acidic food from the stomach. An early deficiency in these neutralizing enzymes can lead to indigestion (acid reflux) and an irritable bowel.

The second "**D**" of vitamin B3 deficiency – **D**ermatitis – is seen as a dry, scaly rash that spreads from the hands/wrists up the arm and feet/ankles up the leg. A red rash shaped like a butterfly across the nose and cheeks can also surface; in keeping with its tell-tale shape, it is called a "butterfly rash."

The third "**D**" of vitamin B3 deficiency – **D**ementia – is a symptom of NAD deficiency because, like the pancreas, nerve cells and brain cells have a huge demand for ATP.

The fourth "**D**" of vitamin B3 deficiency – **D**eath – can in part be explained by increasing acid by-products of glycolysis. When blood becomes too acidic, the heart simply *stops*.

Bottom Line: NAD, from vitamin B3, is needed to make 80% of the ATP that can be made from carbohydrates. ***If NAD deficiency becomes severe, organs will sequentially fail causing symptoms such as diarrhea, dermatitis, dementia and death.***

Chapter 20: Butterflies Everywhere

"Although the world is full of suffering,
it is also full of the overcoming of it.
-Helen Keller

In 1912, a polish chemist named Casimir Funk postulated that there are substances vital to life. His work eventually provided the certain cures for deadly diseases like scurvy (vitamin C deficiency) and pellagra (vitamin B3 deficiency).

What makes these substances vital to life is that they must be consumed from food since human cells cannot make them. Extreme vitamin C and B3 deficiencies can cause death; moderate deficiencies cause a host of diseases that are ascribed various scary-sounding names that can not be reversed with dangerous drugs.

"Vita" means "vital to life". "Amine" designates a nitrogen bond in the chemical make up. It was later discovered that not all of these vital-to-life-amines (vitamins) contain a nitrogen bond.

Vitamins work by moving chemical reactions forward. An example of this is NAD which transports hydrogen to make ATP. A deficiency in vitamin B3, then, results in a slow-down or arrest of the citric acid cycle that NAD normally propels forward.

A myriad of diseases can surface in various organs from moderate to extreme vitamin B3 deficiencies, because every cell in your body needs ATP to function normally.

Doctors generally don't know this. Because they are not taught how to apply nutrition to biochemical science so as to promote or restore cellular health, most physicians do not believe that an overweight and/or sick person is nutrient-starved! Medicine lost its way to offer relief from *symptoms* of disease (dis-ease) rather than curative relief from disease.

In order to preserve life-sustaining organs, the body is designed to "rob Peter to pay Paul." In this light, "Peter" is the skin which has a very low ATP demand and "Paul" is the heart which requires large amounts of ATP for non-stop pumping. As a result, an early sign of vitamin B3 deficiency is a dry, red butterfly rash on the nose and cheeks. This sun-sensitive facial rash may also include the chin and the skin between the eyebrows. Physicians call this "rosacea" which means "red."

If vitamin B3 deficiencies were widespread, one would expect butterfly rashes to be frequent seen…and they are!

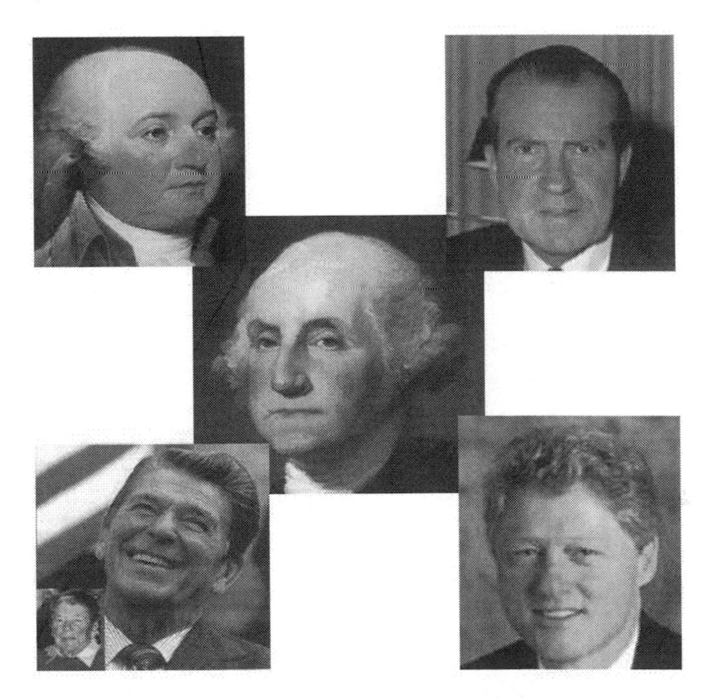

Butterfly rashes commonly afflict the face of overweight people. This is a sign of an NAD-making deficiency; in turn, acetyl-CoA makes fatty acids (fat) instead of ATP. People plagued with chronically-high blood glucose levels often wear the butterfly rash; this signals their NAD-making deficiency and conversion of acetyl-CoA into keto-acids instead of ATP. People complaining of chronic fatigue and sore muscles also display their B3 deficiency mask, revealing their NAD-making deficiency and conversion of acetyl-CoA into lactic acid instead of ATP. Finally, regular alcohol use can trigger a red nose because alcohol depletes vitamin B3.

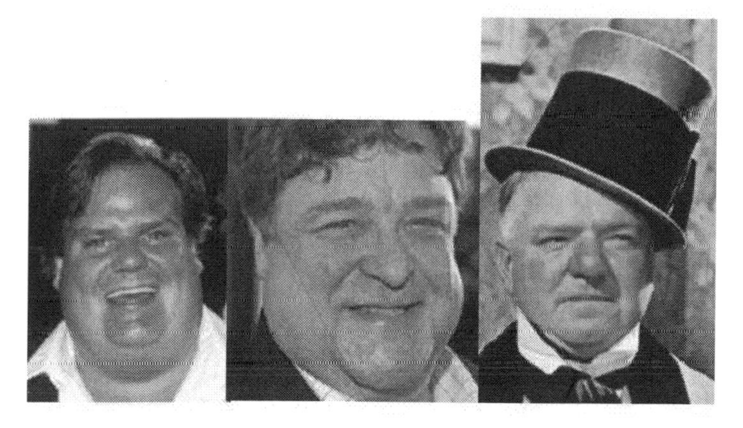

Butterfly rashes are often seen with the same red rash on the forehead, cheeks and chin. These areas represent the skin that covers the oxygen-rich sinuses (the frontal, maxillary and mental sinuses). Oxygen constantly fills these spaces with air breathed through the nose. This skin is more easily damaged by oxygen radicals if sufficient antioxidants such as vitamin C are not part of the daily diet. ***Butterfly rashes, therefore, herald vitamin B3 and vitamin C deficiencies (pellagra and scurvy) – which are no longer diagnosed in western medicine. Both can kill.***

Butterfly rashes are not infrequently seen in people diagnosed with ALS.

Get on the ALS diet and watch your "rosacea" (red") clear up; your doctor will be stumped because physicians largely believe there is no cure for "red"!

A healthy metabolism is the key to a healthy body as well as a healthy butterfly rash-free one. Because a deficiency in NAD backs up the citric acid cycle and forces cells to depend on glycolysis for ATP, one of the early signs of a vitamin B3 deficiency is a loss of energy and an increase in body fat – hence the reason fatigue, fat and butterfly rashes are often found together.

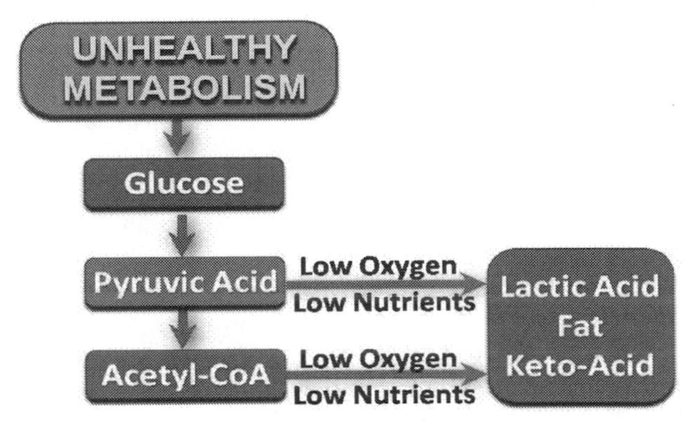

Butterflies, butterflies everywhere; hardly anyone notices the vitamin B3 deficiency right on the end of their nose! What most people do noticc are the varied ill symptoms from a decrease in cellular energy and build up of acid that can be exacerbated by an undiagnosed CWD bacterial infection. ATP, after all, is what makes every cell work. It's the source of energy that allows heart cells to contract and pump your heart. It's the source of energy that allows your nerves to make and transmit chemicals so you can think clearly. It's the source of energy that allows the cells that line your gut to absorb nutrients so the whole process can work in the first place.

Since 80% of the ATP made in any cell comes from vitamin B3 in the form of NAD to deliver hydrogen atoms to the hydrogen dam, without this hydrogen "pressure gradient" to drive the ATP-making process, your batteries become drained. Because a vitamin B3 deficiency leads to an ATP deficiency, every cell is weakened, resulting in diarrhea, a dry rash, dementia and finally death.

Notably, there are two known vitamin deficiencies that can cause death: vitamin B3 and vitamin C. Both often occur together. A vitamin C deficiency also causes blood vessels to become weak and "leaky" – as seen in "spider veins" that are sometimes superimposed on a butterfly rash.

Bottom Line: ***Butterfly rashes, one of the earliest tell-tale signs of a vitamin B3 and vitamin C deficiency, are everywhere…right on the ends of our noses.***

Chapter 21: B3's Are Not Created Equal

"Life is not merely to be alive, but to be well."
-Marcus V. Martial

After the civil war, pellagra plagued the poor of the deep South. A group of prison inmates was selected for an experiment. They were fed the typical diet of the poor in the South. They eventually developed pellagra which proved to be a vitamin B3 deficiency.

Vitamin B3 deficiency is widespread (butterfly faces everywhere) because the form of B3 that the liver preferentially converts to NAD is readily destroyed by modern food processing techniques. Stripping of grains, bleaching, heating and freezing all deplete one of our most valuable resources: the priceless hydrogen-transporting energy-making vitamin B3.

Vitamin B3 comes in two forms: an acid form called *niacin or nicotinic acid* and an amide form called *nicotinamide*. ***The liver preferentially makes NAD from the acid form of B3 and not the amide form of B3*** (references 39 and 40). This is because nicotinic acid contains a chemically-reactive oxygen atom at the site where B3 is converted to NAD. Nicotinamide, on the other hand, has a less chemically-reactive nitrogen atom at the same location.

B3: Nicotinic Acid **B3: Nicotinamide**

O OH N Chemically-reactive

O NH_2 N Chemically-unreactive

NAD

Most B3 supplements as well as the RDA (recommended daily allowance to prevent pellagra) for B3 makes no distinction between B3 as nicotinic acid and B3 as nicotinamide – despite that the latter is poorly converted to NAD by the liver. Perpetuating the error, food and nutrition charts such as those posted by the USDA's on-line information center do not distinguish between food sources with nicotinic acid verses nicotinamide.

To further compound the problem, meats are listed as sources of vitamin B3 – but this is not entirely correct. What is contained in meats is an amino acid called *tryptophan* which cells can convert to niacin, as long as there is sufficient vitamin B6, vitamin B2 and iron in the diet. Vitamin B6 is depleted by use of hormones – which are widely injected into the animal food supply and widely ingested by humans for birth control and hormone replacement therapy. This, in turn, hinders the body's ability to convert tryptophan into vitamin B3. What a mess! Based upon these widely accepted conventions, most nutritionists believe that modern diets are sufficient in vitamin B3 – ***but a plague of butterfly-rashes proves otherwise.***

Nicotinic acid is commonly found in grains, but it is either removed by the stripping of grain hulls (to increase shelf life and decrease the cooking time) or depleted by polishing, processing, storing, refrigerating, freezing and cooking. To accommodate for this, some countries fortify stripped cereals and grains with vitamin B3 – ***but the fortification is with nicotinamide and not nicotinic acid!*** Vitamin supplements also contain B3 in the form of nicotinamide and *not* nicotinic acid. ***Your cells need mostly nicotinic acid and NOT nicotinamide to make NAD – which helps make 80 percent of cellular ATP.***

Nicotinic acid is found mostly in yeast (who eats *that*?), raw seeds (who wants *those*?), raw nuts (you've got to be *kidding* – no roasting?) and raw grains such as rice, bran, barley and wheat (but we strip, polish, pop, puff and cook the B3-life out of those too!).

Nicotinic acid was once the standard for lowering high cholesterol. For decades, it's been known that nicotinic acid (and *not* nicotinamide) lowers cholesterol – albeit by some unknown mechanism. The unknown mechanism remains unknown, nevertheless, because the small but infinitesimally-important detail that the liver preferentially makes NAD from nicotinic acid remains largely unknown.

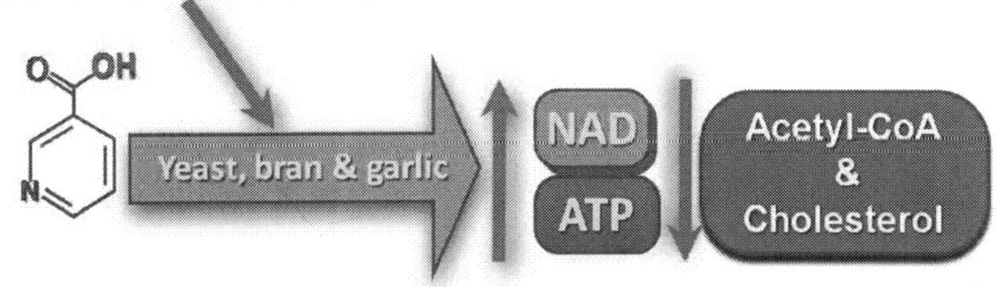

The unknown mechanism of nicotinic acid's cholesterol-lowering effect also remains a mystery because nicotinic acid does not really lower cholesterol – at least not so *directly*. ***This is because NAD propels acetyl-CoA forward into the citric acid cycle to make ATP rather than cholesterol.*** Nicotinic acid, therefore, does *not* lower cholesterol…*it helps makes more ATP from acetyl-CoA*.

Cholesterol, like fat and triglycerides, are made from the building block of acetyl-CoA. Acetyl-CoA fuels the citric acid cycle *if* sufficient nutrients (such as NAD) are on-board to keep the cycle going. If not, then acetyl-CoA will take another metabolic path to make cholesterol, triglycerides, fat or dietary waste acids.

There are few modern food sources rich in vitamin B3 in the form of nicotinic acid. Niacin supplements can cause a temporary but uncomfortable flushing and itch. Supplements in the form of "NAD" or "NADH" tiny tablets are available at most vitamin and health food stores. These are generally well tolerated without any side effects. They are energy boosting, powerful food supplements!

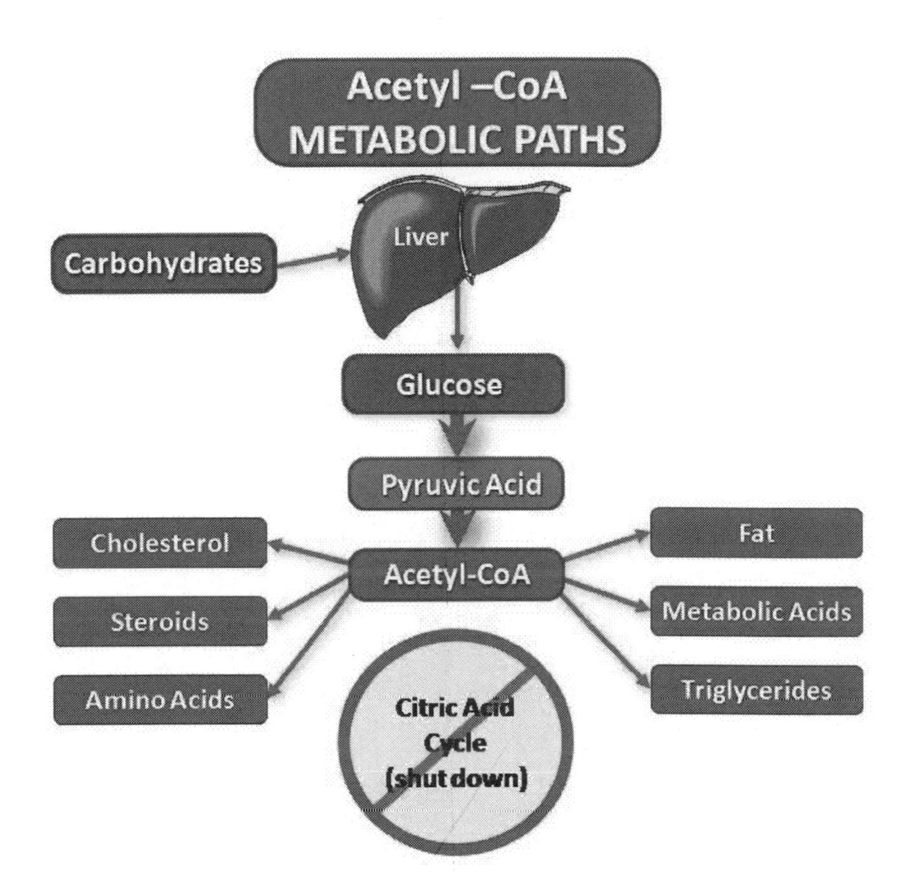

Bottom Line: ***Nicotinic acid, easily destroyed by food processing, is the chemically-reactive form of B3 that the liver preferentially uses to make NAD for ATP production.*** NAD propels acetyl-CoA forward into the citric acid cycle to make ATP, leaving less acetyl-CoA to make fat or acids.

Chapter 22: Body Glue

"Don't dig your grave with your own knife and fork."
-Old English Proverb

Alongside a pandemic of vitamin B3 deficiency – as evidenced by red faces all around us – is widespread vitamin C deficiency. Most mammals make their own vitamin C, but humans and guinea pigs are an exception and must obtain it from food.

Without sufficient vitamin C, the body literally falls apart at the seams. Vitamin C is a key building block of *collagen* which is the "glue" that connects cells, tissues and joints together (*kolla* means *glue*). Collagen literally makes glue, and specialty glues are still made today by boiling collagen from animal skin, bones and tendons.

Collagen is also an important component in the central and peripheral nervous systems. It is no coincidence that both "glia" (from glial cells) and "kolla" mean "glue".

Collagen also lines healthy blood vessels and keeps them smooth and supple. With insufficient vitamin C, the collagen-rich connections between cells are weakened. This lowers the cells' immune defenses and makes it easy for tiny CWD bacteria to invade the inside of cells and cross the blood-brain barrier.

Signs of collagen deficiency are the same as vitamin C deficiency which include frequent infections, skin sores, bleeding gums, easy bruising, nose bleeds, poor wound healing, broken capillaries (often seen over butterfly rashes), leaky blood vessels, hemorrhoids, swollen ankles, thickened skin on elbows and knees (where collagen weakens from repeated bending), fatigue, sore joints and weight gain. Like vitamin B3 deficiency, an uncorrected vitamin C deficiency can kill.

Like vitamin B3, vitamin C is also key to a lean and healthy body for two reasons: One, collagen makes strong cells (where metabolism takes place) and two, vitamin C helps to make *carnitine*, which is a transport molecule that shuttles fat into cells for oxidation by the citric acid cycle.

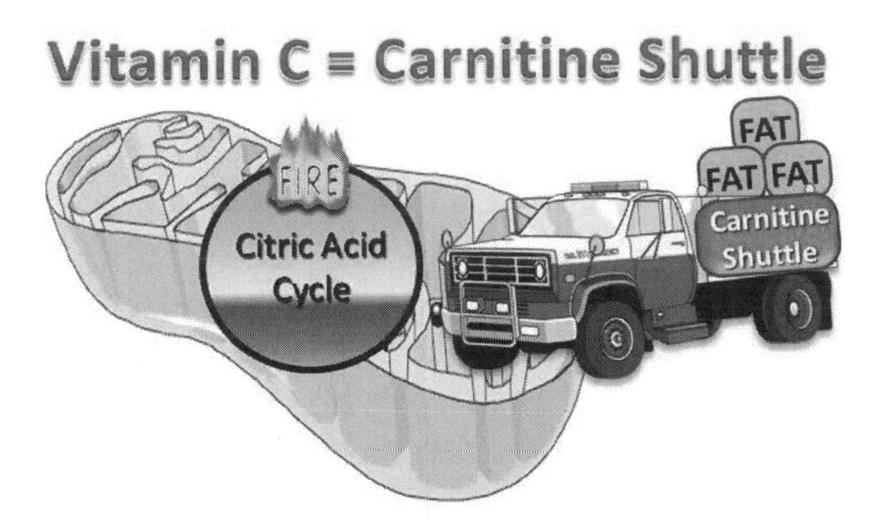

Need to strengthen cells, boost the immune system and/or lose fat? Then get on board the Carnitine Shuttle and load up on vitamin C! But don't go buying ready-made pasteurized juices supposedly rich in vitamin C because vitamin C is *extremely* sensitive to heating – even more so than nicotinic acid – and it is quickly destroyed by pasteurization.

Four carbohydrates have been found to significantly decrease the risk of infection and cardiovascular disease: apples, tomatoes, onions and broccoli. All are rich in vitamin C.

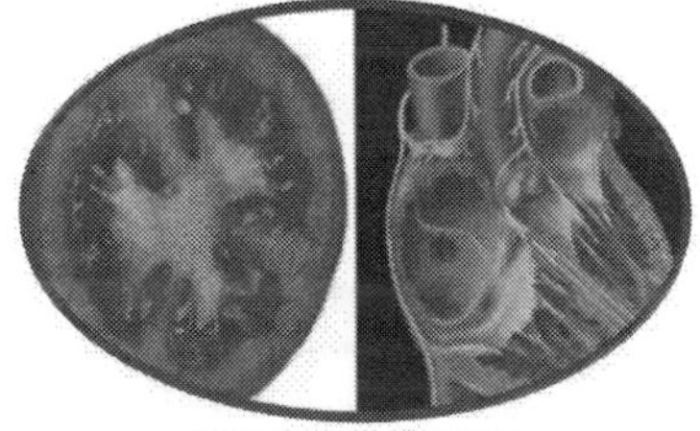

Bottom Line: Vitamin C is vital for two important molecules that start with "C". ***Collagen is the glue that holds cells together, and carnitine is the shuttle for transporting fat into cells for oxidation into ATP.*** Vitamin C keeps you glued and burns the acids and fat!

Chapter 23: Eat More, Not Less

"Without health, there is no point. To anything."
-Everett Mámor

To conquer ALS and follow Hippocrates' advice ("Let food be your medicine") two things are required:

1. A basic understanding of how food converts to energy.
2. A desire to change old habits to bring the science to life.

How, then, shall we eat? It is cosmically simple! Eat to make maximum hydrogen and ATP which is the universal fuel for every cell in a body.

Do NOT count calories. Rather, consider the ATP (hydrogen) that a food can make! Non-nutritious food can only turn to acid and fat – no matter how few calories of it you eat. Eat only a small amount of dead calories and you will slowly lose more of your health and/or slowly gain fat.

Stop counting calories of food that can not oxidize.

Eat more and not less of foods that make ATP. Cells need lots of nutrients and oxygen-rich slightly basic water that promote oxidation. Foods, then, should be selected based upon their content of the following big three energy-making nutrients:

1. Vitamin C (citrus, tomatoes, onions,broccoli and squash)
2. Malic Acid (apples)
3. Nicotinic Acid

Vitamin C fortifies cells (the hydrogen energy dam can't function very well if it's falling apart at the seams) and makes carnitine for burning excess fat. Malic acid and nicotinic acid directly fuel the citric acid cycle. Citrus fruits rich in vitamin C are also high in citric acid which directly ignites the citric acid cycle.

In what has come to be known as the "acid-alkaline diet", some nutritionists recommend avoiding "acidic" carbs like citrus fruits in favor of alkaline fruits like melons. This is a completely WRONG concept. The acidity of a carbohydrate does NOT make body water acidic. It is the nutrients in carbs that determines whether or not they will fully oxidize into hydrogen and carbon dioxide – or acid wastes.

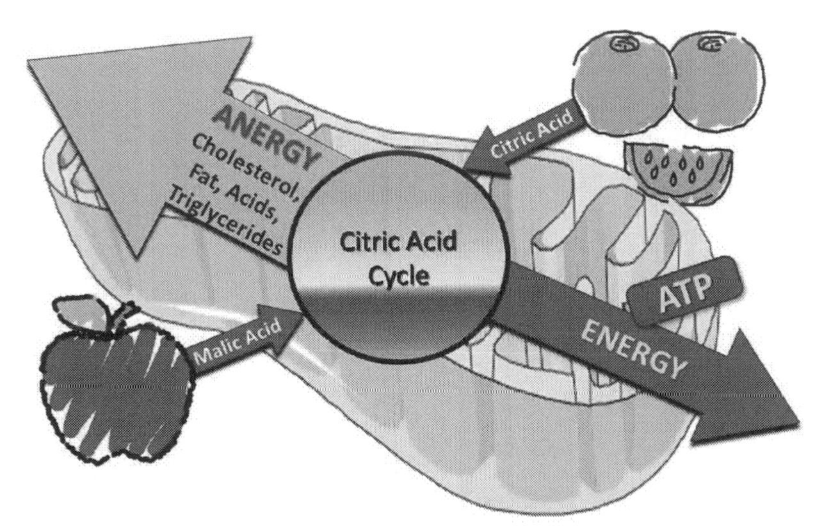

The opposite of energy is anergy. Any food that pushes the citric acid forward promotes energy (ATP) and prevents anergy (fat). Foods that make energy also satisfy the hunger center in the brain and stave off the appetite.

A vicious cycle continues when foods are consumed that do not make energy/ATP. When oxidation slows, the brain stimulates hunger cravings specifically for *carbohydrates*, because the brain can only function well with energy made from carbohydrates (rather than protein or fat). Brain cells have a high demand for energy; this organ is, after all, your central processing unit and it requires a constant ATP pool to make and send neurotransmitters through a complex array of nerves.

Low ATP triggers the hunger center in the brain which releases acid in your stomach, saliva in your mouth and stirs up your hunger pangs.

Calorie-counting or avoiding acidic foods reflects a complete absence of knowledge about carbohydrate oxidation. Calories are calculated experimentally by completely burning a food into ash and measuring the heat. The gross assumption is that the food will completely oxidize (burn) into hydrogen inside cells. THAT IS SO WRONG! You can eat 500 calories per day of nutrient deficient food and still gain weight or become ill if the food doesn't completely oxidize. And the fact of the matter is that processed carbohydrates that can sit on shelves indefinitely CAN'T oxidize because they are dead, depleted, deficient – pick a word – of nutrients.

Being healthy is not about how many calories you eat or don't eat; it's about whether or not the food you eat contains the nutrients to support the metabolic process of oxidizing it into hydrogen and converting it into ATP.

Being thin does not equate to health. You can be thin and even have low blood cholesterol – when inside your cells and tissues are pools of CWD parasites converting acetyl-CoA into pyruvic acid and gobbling up fat and cholesterol from cell membranes and nerves.

Because vitamins like B3 and C are water-soluble, the body cannot store them. Therefore, any excess B and C vitamins exit the body via the water (urine). These nutrients must therefore be ingested *daily*. You can starve yourself and be lean – or even exercise constantly and look thin – and yet be starved and infected at the cellular level if these vitamins are lacking.

The only way to conquer ALS and then maintain your health is to *never* count calories. ***If you're eating a nutrient-poor food that***

can't completely oxidize into hydrogen, you shouldn't eat it in the first place! It isn't a life-propelling, energy-promoting food. IT ISN'T FOOD! If you need to count calories because too much will make you fat, then that food makes anergy and not energy. DON'T EAT IT! Run away from the table! That food will only make you into two four-letter-words: ACID and SICK.

No food is more nutritious and satisfying than the apple. The more apples you eat, the more full you will feel, the more healthy and energized you will become and, if overweight, the more fat you will lose – as long as you don't also stuff your cells with anergy-making, man-manipulated carbohydrates to offset the work of the amazing apple.

While apples are rich in vitamin C, the secret nutrient for their health-promoting effect is *malic acid* which directly fuels the citric acid cycle:

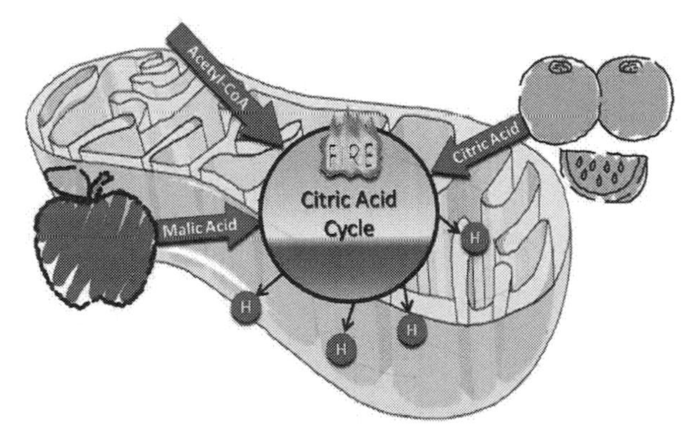

This stoking of the energy cycle by malic acid in apples allows more acetyl-CoA (from carbohydrate foods or fat) to combine with the oxidation product of malic acid to make citric acid which can enter into the citric acid cycle…and on and on the hydrogen-to-ATP-making cycle goes, satisfying your brain and shutting down your appetite.

A quick way to prepare raw apples is spiral-sliced and cored with an apple peeler. This tool slices and cores with a simple spear of an apple and turn of a handle. To prevent the slices from turning brown (vitamin C oxidizes very quickly when exposed to air), simply dip the apple slices in a bowl of fresh-squeezed orange juice or juice of any citrus fruit (citric acid is a natural preservative). Eat as many of these as you want throughout the day and enjoy restoring your body slowly back to health without a wince of a hunger pang.

Diced or mashed apples cooked in a bit of water and flavored with cinnamon and stevia are acceptable – but the heat will

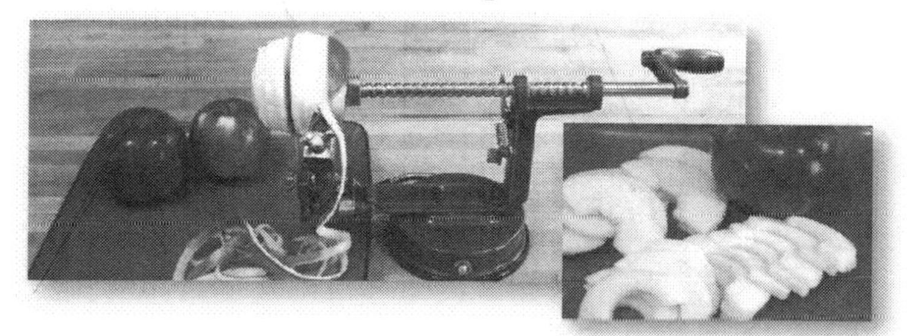

destroy some of the nutrients. If you don't have much time for food preparation, store bought sugar-free apple sauce will still increase your metabolism but there's no equal substitute for raw apples.

One of the best ways to fuel your cells with six apples and six oranges once or twice a day is to juice them. Forget any store bought juice that's been heated by pasteurization; there is little to no natural vitamin C left in the juice, no matter how much the manufacturer claims otherwise. ***Vitamin C is extremely temperature-sensitive.*** For this reason, store bought pasteurized fruit juice will make anergy instead of ATP. Even fresh juice made at home will lose some potency after two days of refrigeration.

If you've suffered from irregularity, that is a sign that the cells lining the small intestine lack the energy to efficiently digest and propel food forward. Small intestinal cells are the first to suffer from nutrient deficiency; on the other hand, they are the first to recover! Vitamin C rich foods and fresh juice will normalize bowel function – sometimes too well with temporary diarrhea. When balanced, regular (daily) bowel movements of well-formed floating stool will follow. This is a sign of health restoration! When the intestinal cells are satisfied, nutrients will be shared with the rest of the body. You will then enjoy regularity as long as the ALS diet is your mainstay.

Another sign that intestinal cells are becoming healthy again is a change from a white-coated tongue (damaged cells) to a normal pink-red tongue without fissures. The tongue, after all, is the start of the digestive tract!

Second to the apple, the next nutrient-loaded carbohydrate for revving up the citric acid cycle is the tomato. Despite the vitamin C in tomatoes is heat-sensitive, other important nutrients such as lycopenes are not. ***Raw or cooked, you can literally stuff yourself with tomatoes and all you will do is maintain your optimal weight and enjoy restored health.***

The third super-fuel food is the onion – rich in vitamin C and minerals that propel ATP production forward. Like apples, the more RAW onions you eat the more better health you will enjoy. Stir-fried onions mixed with canned stewed tomatoes and topped with raw diced sweet onion are at the top of the list of power-meals.

The fourth vitamin C-rich food group is the squash family: summer squash, zucchini, butternut squash, acorn squash and

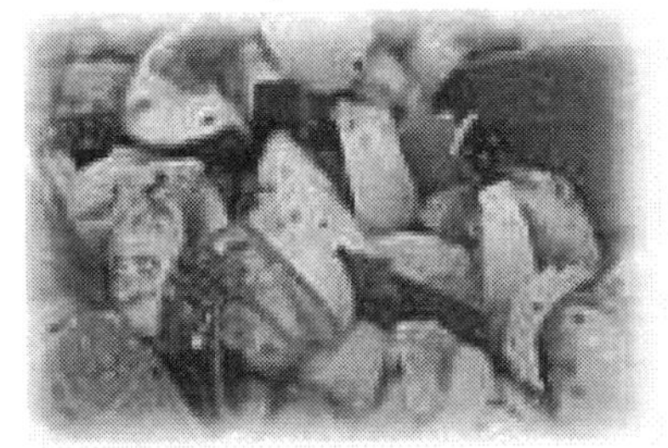

cucumber. Cooked or raw, the more you eat the better you will feel – but the less cooked the better. Combining the last three food groups makes a nice dish of stewed tomatoes, onions and zucchini.

When you're full, stop eating. When you're hungry again, eat as much as you want! In time, your body will be nagging you for more vitamin C rich carbohydrates (mainly raw fruits and vegetables). The desire for dead foods will be vanquished. Be patient and watch as your cells' health is restored and your body water returned to a normal oxygen-rich pH. As this happens, you will notice that activities that used to rob you of breath and energy are becoming more easy!

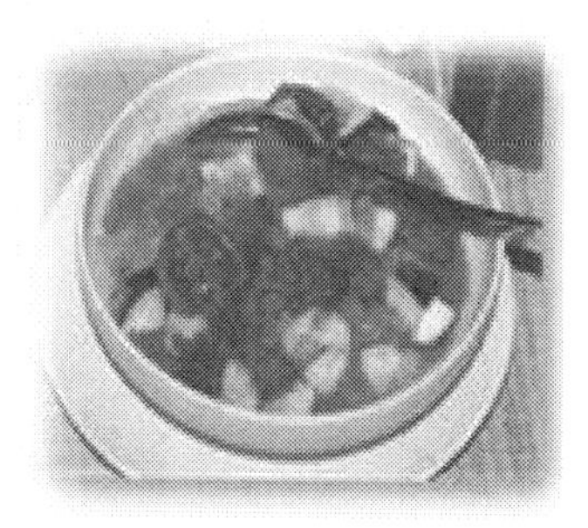

Remember, basic water has more oxygen. When cells that make up tissues and organs have more oxygen, so do you! The reason you breathe in the first place is to obtain oxygen for cellular oxidation. Oxygen is the final "nutrient" used up in the process of converting hydrogen into ATP; carbon dioxide is the by-product that you breathe out. If you used to be a shallow breather, when oxidation is fired up you may notice that you naturally take deep, full breaths. Increased stamina and "breath" are signs that cellular health is being restored.

Most all fruits and vegetables contain some amount of vitamin C, but some have more than others. More excellent sources of vitamin C include cabbage, peppers, cauliflower, green beans, broccoli, leafy greens, sweet potatoes, cantaloupe, strawberries, blueberries and watermelon. Eat up!

Nicotinic acid – the building block of NAD for making 80% of your potential energy – is rich in raw nuts, raw seeds and mushrooms (it is found in all grains but destroyed by milling and heating). Nicotinic acid is so quickly ruined by food-processing that, short of eating *raw* nuts and seeds (roasting destroys B vitamins), it is best supplemented with a vitamin supplement in the form of NAD or NADH.

Nicotinic acid is also high in coffee (highest in instant coffee) and tobacco – so while I don't recommend either product, now you know why so many people addicted to coffee and cigarettes have trouble with fatigue and fat when they kick the habit.

Final thought: There is another fruit like the amazing apple that is rich in malic acid and vitamin C – grapes! Many people avoid grapes because they are sweet and so they think the natural sugar will make them fat. Now you know better! Eat 'em – in bunches with apples!

This is not a mix and match diet. A little dead food mixed with good food will still kill you. Dead food, fast food and snack food must be gone forever.

Bottom Line: ***Carbohydrates rich in vitamin C, malic acid and nicotinic acid power the energy cycle of cells so effectively, that more they are eaten the more ATP is made and the more excess fatty acid is burned.*** These include: apples, tomatoes, onions and squash. Oh yes, and grapes.

Chapter 24: Forks in the Road

"While we can't control all that happens to us, we can control what happens inside us."
-Ben Franklin

Soda is without doubt one of the worst poisons that someone can pour down his or her throat. The acidity chokes the life out of oxidative metabolism and turns cells into acid cesspools. When oxidation is hindered, cells default to the ancient mechanism of metabolism: glycolysis. Glycolysis is the simplest method of metabolism for both the primordial single-celled microbe like Chlamydia pneumoniae and any oxygen-deficient human cell.

When cells are low on oxygen – such as the muscle cells of a marathoner – the cells will be blocked from oxidation and resort to glycolysis. Due to the lack of cellular oxygen, the citric acid cycle is shut down, resulting in a build up of lactic acid which hurts. After the race, and the athlete rests for a few days days; oxidation resumes and lactic acid is oxidized into hydrogen. Life and limbs feel normal again.

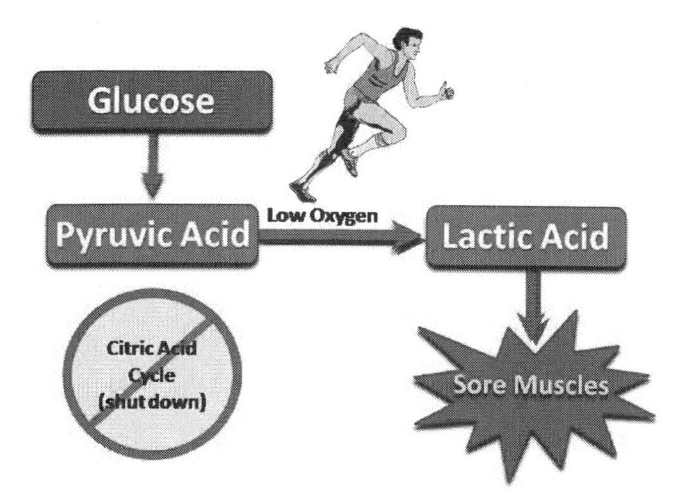

Like oxygen deprivation from exercise (or even smoking), a host of ill effects occur when cells are deprived of certain nutrients. ***A lack of oxygen is not the only deficiency to hinder oxidation and cause a painful build up of lactic acid in muscle.*** A closer look will get to the fat and acid of the matter.

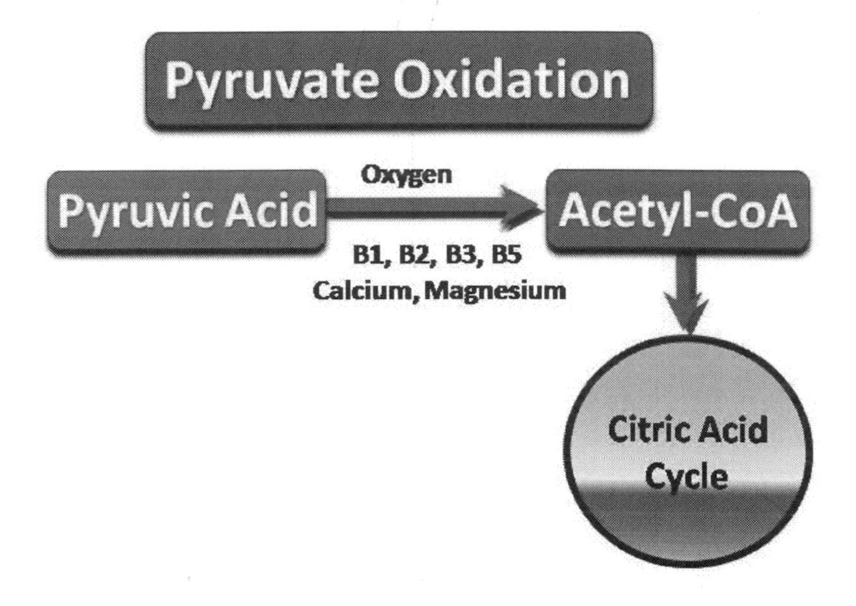

The first step of metabolism, or glycolysis, takes place inside cell water. The product of glycolysis is pyruvic acid which enters the mitochondria where it is oxidized into acetyl-CoA. This is called *pyruvate oxidation* and is the first step of oxidation.

What acetyl-CoA makes at this juncture determines whether you are healthy or sick because acetyl-CoA is the link between glycolysis and oxidation.

Pyruvate oxidation, or the making of acetyl-CoA, requires an enzyme called *pyruvate dehydrogenase complex* (enzymes stimulate chemical reactions). Molecules abbreviated as “TPP” and “FAD” are part of this enzyme complex.

What is lost in translation in medical school biochemistry books is that TPP is made from vitamin B1 and FAD is made from vitamin B2! The molecule acetyl-CoA is even derived from vitamin B5 – and so B5 must be available as well as B1 and B2 for any of this to work. Also, for pyruvate oxidation to be complete, a supply of NAD (from vitamin B3), magnesium and calcium must all be present within the mitochondria.

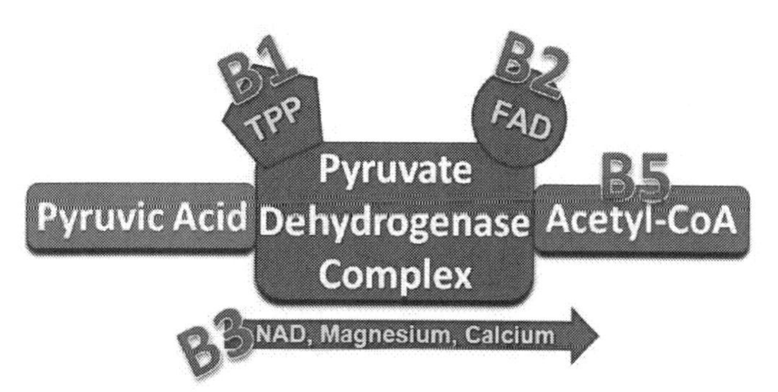

Both nutrient (vitamins and minerals) and oxygen deficiencies can shut down oxidation via the citric acid cycle!

No acetyl-CoA means no citric acid cycle which means no oxidation of glucose – and a deficiency in vitamins B1, B2, B3 and B5 and/or a deficiency in the minerals magnesium and calcium can all hinder the making of acetyl-CoA which is needed to make ATP. No wonder we see so many red noses! And, because these B-vitamins are water-soluble, they cannot be stored up in the tissues but most be obtained every day from carbohydrate foods. Nutrient-deficient food, if even oxidized to acetyl-CoA, can be doomed to eviction from the ATP-making mitochondria if it can't burn in the citric acid cycle.

Many people with symptoms of oxidation deficiency such as chronic fatigue and sore, stiff muscles are sometimes advised by their physicians to exercise. While exercise certainly increases delivery of oxygen to cells and would seem to enhance oxidation, without replacing the vitamin and mineral deficiencies that can also block oxidation, exercise will inevitably exacerbate symptoms of fatigue and pain as more and more metabolic acid

by-products such as lactic acid build up in tissues. This will also serve to feed acid-loving unwanted microbes.
Insulin also pushes this reaction forward. The mechanisms of insulin are not well-understood, but high levels of glucose in the blood – called type 2 diabetes – clearly involves much more than a "resistance to the action of insulin" which is the mantra of western medicine. The successful oxidation of pyruvate into acetyl-CoA is dependent not only on insulin but on many minerals and B-vitamins that are stripped in modern foods. Notably, physicians in India often prescribe multi-B vitamins and magnesium to type 2 diabetics.

Once acetyl-CoA is made, a chemical reaction traps it inside the mitochondria to make ATP. If insufficient nutrients are in the mitochondria to oxidize acetyl-CoA, then acetyl-CoA is transported out of the mitochondria by another chemical reaction called the C*itrate Shuttle*. In the process of moving acetyl-CoA out of the mitochondria back into the cell water, vitamin B3 is also shuttled out of the mitochondria in the form of NADP, which is used to make fatty acids in the cell water.

Rejected from the ATP-making process, acetyl-CoA now faces a biochemical fork-in-the-road, one of which is making acid. Back in the cell water, acetyl-CoA can make the following potentially health-destroying molecules:

1. Acetyl-CoA molecules combine as the first step to make **CHOLESTEROL**.
2. Acetyl-CoA joins with glycerol to make **TRIGLYCERIDES**.
3. Acetyl-CoA makes **FAT**.
4. Acetyl-CoA from fat makes **ACID**.

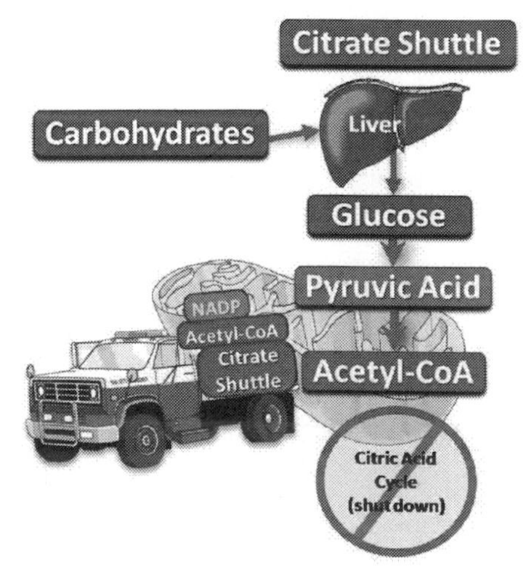

While the supply of acetyl-CoA is what drives the citric acid cycle inside the mitochondria of cells, a lack of B vitamins, magnesium and calcium can result in the eviction of acetyl-CoA from the ATP-making process. ***Evicted acetyl-CoA, then, must make an alternative acidic molecule for storage.***

Where there is one vitamin deficiency there is usually a multitude of deficiencies. If a vitamin C deficiency is also brewing inside cells, then cells and tissues will be lacking the collagen that holds cells and tissues tightly together to help ward off infections; frequent colds and chronic infections are the lot. Two acetyl-CoA molecules can start a chain reaction that makes cholesterol to repair damaged cells, myelin and blood vessels from chronic infections of cholesterol-robbing CWD microbes like Chlamydia pneumoniae. When the citric acid cycle is shut down, acetyl-CoA can also make acids called *ketone bodies* that provide an alternative (albeit inferior) energy source for the brain. Finally, if there is no crisis such as cellular damage or a need for alternative energy for the brain to function, acetyl-CoA can make fat and triglycerides which can later be reconverted into acetyl-CoA for re-entry into the mitochondria for oxidation into ATP – if a cell's nutritional status so permits.

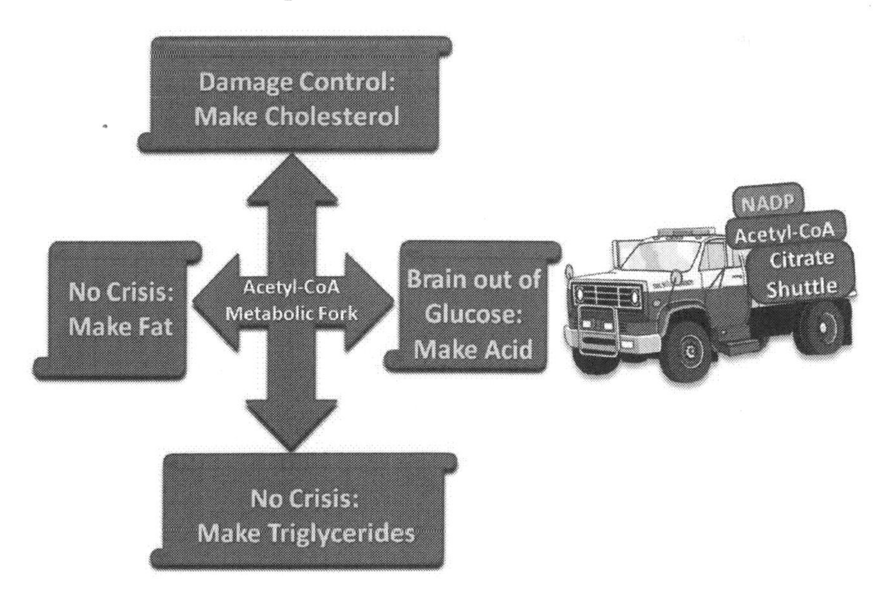

If you have read this far, by now you know that true proven science and common sense mix very well. Money, drugs and medicine do not.

Bottom Line: ***The nutrients present in carbohydrates determine whether acetyl-CoA will enter the citric acid cycle and make energy or be evicted into the cell water to make acid, cholesterol, fat or triglycerides.***

Chapter 25: Do the Shuttle

"Live long and prosper."
-Dr. Spock

There are three metabolic transport systems awaiting delivery of every carbohydrate morsel that enters your mouth: the Citrate Shuttle, the Citric Acid Cycle and the Carnitine Shuttle. The first delivers ill health, the second maintains metabolic health and the third promotes health restoration.

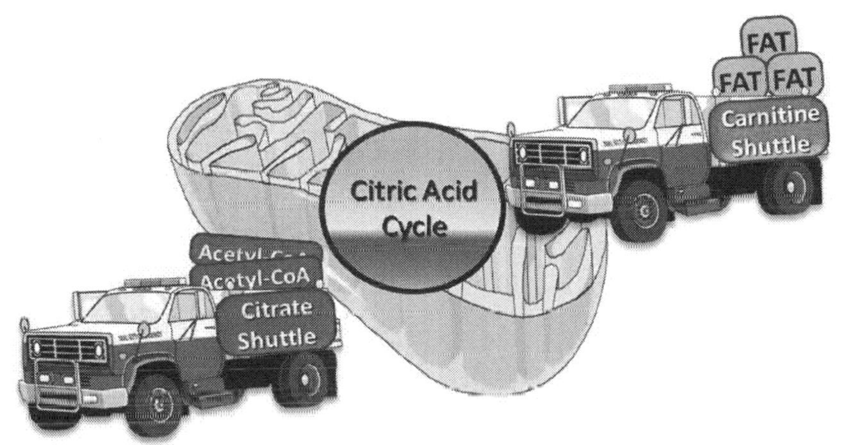

Acetyl-CoA is either being shuttled to the mitochondria to be burned, or it is being shuttled away from the mitochondria into the cell water to make fat for storage or to be converted into another molecule.

If you think that you can simply skip this carbohydrate shuttle system by eating more protein, then think again. While eating more protein will circumvent fat gain (the Citrate Shuttle), your cells will be robbed of the nutrients needed to promote health via the Citric Acid Cycle because most life-supporting vitamins and hydrogen atoms are found in carbohydrates – *not protein*. Also, protein must be filtered by millions of tiny filters in the kidney and thus taxes the kidneys. Finally, protein metabolizes into amino *acids* which pushes water pH in the wrong direction.

If you have been diagnosed with ALS and are thin or lean, press on your outer elbow, knee and ankle joints, chest wall, shoulder blades and hip girdle. If it hurts, those are dietary acids built up in the tender sheathes of tendon that connect muscle to bone. Acids hurt! When those tender spots begin to hurt less and you generally feel better, cellular health is being restored.

There is no way to avoid the carbohydrate shuttle. You may circumvent it for a season but sooner or later your brain, which can only function optimally on carbs, is going to be *screaming* at you to eat carbohydrates. These automatic (hard-wired) cravings from your central processing unit will eventually overcome your willful choice of an alternative energy source such as a high protein diet.

Avoiding the carbohydrate shuttle, in the end, only results in confronting an endless yo-yo of health gain and health loss, up and down and up and down and with nowhere to go but up and down. So do the shuttle and face reality. It makes much more biochemical sense!

Choosing the correct carbohydrate shuttle means choosing the route to the fire instead of away from it. Remember, it is all those peanut-shaped swimming pools called mitochondria that are your cells' energy furnaces. If they are stocked with the nutrients to completely oxidize carbohydrates, then the final products will be carbon dioxide (exhaled from the lungs), hydrogen (made into energy as ATP), water (discharged through the urinary tract) and heat (a normal 98.6°F body-temperature).

If you find yourself feeling cold when most everyone else is warm or comfortable, that is another sign that your metabolism is dysfunctional. When you're on-target with the ALS diet and your mitochondria are spewing out ATP, you will generally feel warmer and more cold tolerant.

The citric acid cycle inside mitochondria is like fire in a wood-burning furnace. Wood is a carbohydrate and when it burns (oxidizes) it makes energy and heat. The carbohydrates you eat also oxidize (burn) to make energy and heat. Like a wood-burning fire, oxidation is a chemical process that requires three things: oxygen, heat (98.6°F) and fuel (nutrient-rich carbohydrates).

Without one of these elements a fire simply cannot start or continue. Vitamins and minerals from the ALS diet are your fuel.

Some people think that eating a few large meals in a day slows down the metabolism and that the key to turning up one's metabolism is to eat more frequent and smaller meals. Others believe that fasting will slow down one's metabolism, as the endocrine system readjusts to preserve energy in a starvation mode. None of these ideas make one lick of biochemical sense.

Oxidation is either on, off or in between. If you put moist wood into a furnace, it might burn for awhile and then burn out; oxidation will be off. Throw some fuel-oil on the wood and light it again, and it will burn; oxidation will be on. In between "on and off" can be a slow smoldering fire that is on its way out.

Cooked, processed carbohydrates are like wet wood. ***It is not the calories in a carbohydrate that make it a fuel for your mitochondrial fires, it is the nutrients within the carbohydrates you eat that make food a good fuel or bad fuel for the fire.*** Wet, cooked food is like wet wood – unsuitable for sustainable combustion because wet, cooked and processed food

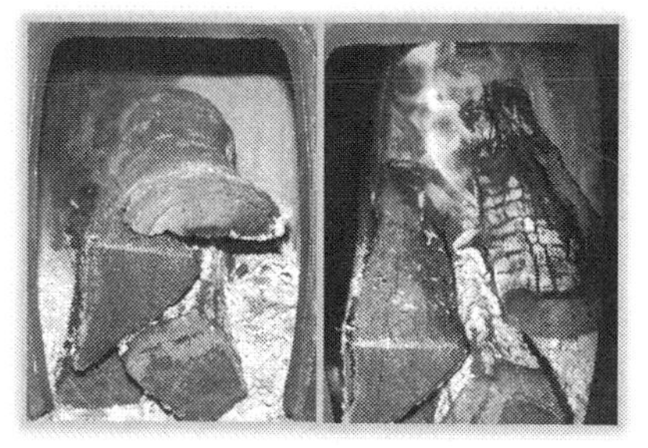

is nutrient-deficient food. It is an incompletely-combustible fuel no matter how few calories of it you eat.

Wet food is dead food just like wet wood is dead wood.

Your mitochondria are persnickety: they simply don't want a bunch of dead, wet or partially burned wood left inside their furnaces – and so enters the Citrate Shuttle to dump the partially-combusted acetyl-CoA back into the cell water. "GET OUT!" is the standing order. "Burn, or ship out!"

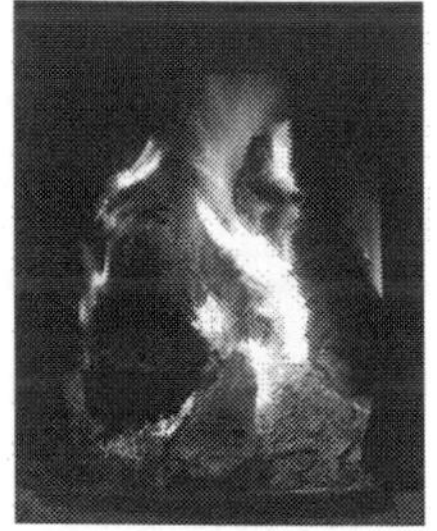

Now, if you want to get on the health promoting acid burning shuttle rather than try to circumvent biochemical law, then get on the Carnitine Shuttle. This is where you turn your mitochondria furnaces to the "on" and FULL BLAST oxidation mode.

Carnitine, you may recall, is made from Vitamin C. Vitamin C, like the B-vitamins, cannot be made or stored inside cells. There are no vitamin B and vitamin C storehouses in your cells; you either obtain these vitamins with every bite of food you eat, or you don't. Because these vitamins are water-soluble, they filter through the kidney into the urine (your "water").
Dissolved vitamin B2, or riboflavin, turns water bright orange-yellow. Some physicians like to joke that vitamins only make "expensive urine." Orange urine is not a sign of "wasted" vitamins. It is simply the visible evidence of water-soluble B2. It is also proof that vitamins readily absorbed are also readily lost. They must be constantly consumed.

So, because vitamin C is water-soluble and temperature-sensitive, if you want to take the Carnitine Shuttle every day then you will need lots of fresh sources of vitamin C every day. ***Carnitine is what shuttles fat (solid waste dietary acid) and liquid waste dietary acid stored in tissues into the mitochondrial furnaces for conversion into ATP.*** Chlamydia pneumoniae hates the Carnitine shuttle.

Along with vitamin C, you will need daily fresh foods rich in vitamins B1, B2, B3 (as nicotinic acid), B5, magnesium and calcium. Carnitine helps to transfer the solid waste acid (called "fat" which is made from fatty acids) and other liquid dietary acids into the fire of the mitochondria. The B-vitamins and minerals will serve to help burn it up (oxidation).

Every food choice should be made so as to select nutrients that support the Carnitine Shuttle and the Citric Acid Cycle.

Avoid foods that stimulate the Citrate shuttle. Your life and health depend on it!

Bottom Line: ***Some things in life cannot be avoided, and the carbohydrate shuttle is one of them.*** Carbohydrates, in the form of acetyl-CoA, are either being shuttled *to* or away *from* the mitochondrial energy furnaces. The direction simply depends on the food one chooses to eat.

Chapter 26: Keep the Fire Burning

"It's much easier to ride the horse in the direction he's going."
-Werner Erhard

If you have been diagnosed with ALS *and* type-2 diabetes, the two are not mutually exclusive; both conditions of dis-ease (lost ease) can be conquered by restoring metabolic health. This chapter offers more food for thought in conquering both ALS and diabetes.

If a fire in your fireplace isn't burning very well, it makes little sense to keep pushing logs into the fireplace, simply because you want a smaller stockpile of logs in your wood shed. Likewise, if the mitochondria in your cells are not oxidizing glucose very well, it makes little sense to take drugs that will push more glucose into your cells, simply because you want less glucose in your blood.

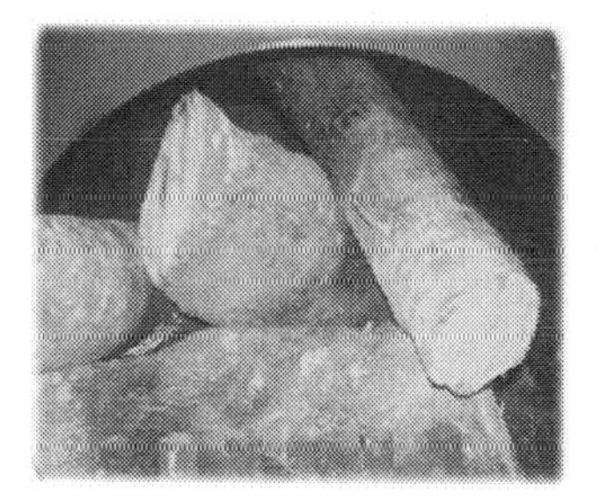

Like a plugged drain backs up water in a sink, glucose that is poorly oxidizing within cells begins to back up blood glucose that normally enters cells to oxidize into ATP. The most popular drugs for type-2 diabetes do not help cells to oxidize glucose. Rather, they work by forcing glucose out of the blood into cells. It makes the numbers of a blood test look better, but it doesn't fix the problem. Because the mitochondria aren't oxidizing glucose effectively, in time more and more of the same drug is required to get the same effect to lower blood glucose.

In a similar vein, if a fire isn't burning very well, it takes more and more effort to jam more logs into the same fireplace.

Type-2 diabetes is described as a "metabolic disorder" but the pill-form pharmaceutical drugs do not restore metabolic health. They are more like chemical "hat tricks" to make blood lab reports look better which only makes your doctor *think* that he's done some good.

What if you purchased a car thinking that the engine had little wear when the truth of the matter was that the odometer had been disconnected to make the numbers look good? You were fooled! It is no difference with drugs that simply shift molecules from the blood into cells. While this may prevent some of the problems that elevated blood glucose can cause to cells that line the blood vessels, the problem is shifted to other tissue cell types.

Everything in nature follows a course that "relieves itself" from high pressure to low pressure – a downhill gradient, if you will. Movement is often stopped or slowed, then, when a gradient has been blocked. For example, our filled stomachs don't accommodate more food until emptied; our brains may block another new concept until the one just presented to it has been processed; without an opportunity to relieve a full bladder, we decline another drink.

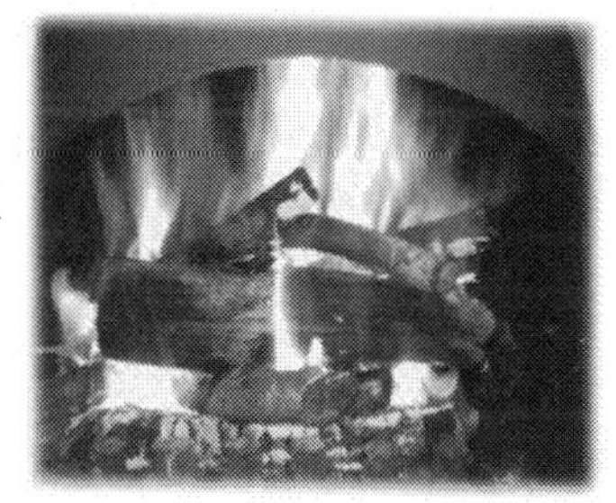

Just as a fireplace with a well oxygenated hot fire will quickly burn more logs thrown onto the grate, so will nutrient-enriched mitochondria efficiently oxidize glucose and make room for more glucose to enter cells from the blood.

Physicians are taught that type-2 diabetes is a "metabolic disorder" due to cells having become "insulin-resistant." They learn that insulin is like a key that opens up insulin receptors on cell membranes so that glucose can enter the cell. Diabetic drugs are designed to increase the sensitivity of insulin receptors so that glucose can more easily transit through "insulin resistant" cell membranes. Because drug companies fund drug research in most every medical school, they influence paradigms and protocols,

right or wrong, that favor widespread use of their drugs.
By design or willful ignorance, physicians are not taught how to apply nutrition to oxidative metabolism; they therefore don't have a clue how to correct a glucose metabolizing disorder. This ignorance is reflected in bad advice such as avoiding certain foods that help correct the problem – and widespread use of drugs that fix little more than numbers on lab results.

Physicians are also taught that people with elevated body fat are at high risk for insulin resistance. This is an observation of symptoms, *not cause*. Insulin resistance and increased body fat go hand-in-hand.

A failing carbohydrate metabolism due to multiple nutrient deficiencies results in increased dietary waste acids, increased body fat and, in time if not corrected, elevated blood glucose – NOT the other way around. In time, cells with nutrient-depleted mitochondria become resistant to glucose, because poorly oxidized acetyl-CoA is evicted from mitochondria via the Citrate Shuttle to make fatty acids. Nutrient depleted cells, stuffed with partly oxidized glucose in the form of acetyl-CoA, resist entrance to more glucose from the blood. ***Fix the fire, and then the cell will receive more "wood" (glucose) to burn.***

Elevated Blood Glucose:

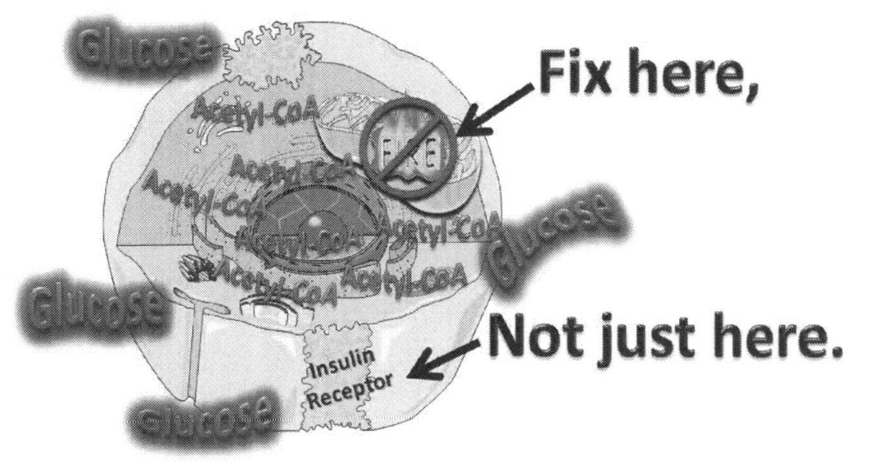

Cell membranes become resistant to insulin because the glucose burning machinery is broken and the chocolate candies on the conveyer belt are backing up. Insulin resistance (glucose resistance) in this light, then, is simply a symptom of poor oxidation, *and not the cause*. Drugs that stuff more chocolate candies on the conveyer belt are nonsense; they make no sense!

Persistently elevated blood glucose is due to mitochondrial resistance to glucose (cause) rather than cell membrane resistance to glucose (a symptom of the cause).

Put another way that is cosmically simple: Elevated blood glucose is a sign that the CITRATE SHUTTLE (chapter 25) rather than the CITRIC ACID CYCLE is activated.

Treating the problem, then, is found in restoring carbohydrate oxidation within mitochondria and not simply in pushing more glucose into cells with drugs. Because type-2 diabetes is a metabolic disorder, it is a dysfunction of the mitochondria because this is where oxidation of glucose occurs! One of the symptoms of dysfunctional mitochondria is cell membrane resistance to more glucose. Glucose then backs up in the blood.

Think of this as a husband shutting his office door to a bickering wife; he has simply become resistant to hearing any more words from her until he can process what has already been dished out. This explains why some type-2 diabetics are able to normalize their blood glucose levels with nutrients that support carbohydrate oxidation.

Before prescribing drugs that help push glucose out of blood into cells, most physicians will first recommend dietary changes to patients with borderline abnormal blood glucose levels; some of this advice, however, completely derails success. Patients are often advised, for example, to eat less "sugary" fruits which are chock-full of malic acid, citric acid, vitamin C and the minerals so necessary for normalizing metabolism. No physician would recommend raw honey to a diabetic, but raw honey is so packed with nutrients to jump-start the citric acid cycle, that one teaspoon of raw honey can lower blood glucose like 10 units of insulin (reference 41)!

Like raw honey, one of the most potent health tonics for lowering elevated blood glucose is apple cider vinegar diluted in water or mixed in fresh-squeezed apple juice.

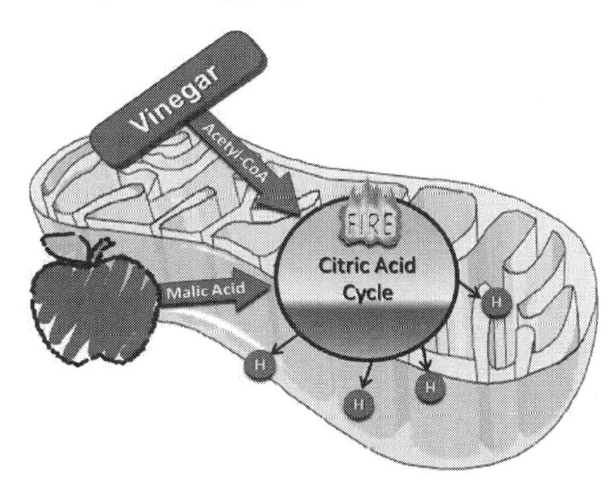

Notably, raw honey helps "feed" the good bacteria in the gut; this serves to neutralize overpopulation of toxin-making CWD lifeforms in the gut. For many years now, an association has been found with H. pylori infection and elevated blood glucose. Statin use has also increased the risk of type 2 diabetes. Natural steps, therefore, to decrease CWD toxins and food based mycotoxins serves to help normalize blood sugar levels by pushing oxidation forward (remember, CWD's in cells preferentially use glycolysis which serves to engage the citrate shuttle). Raw honey and yogurt with live active probiotic cultures are potent medicines for people with elevated blood glucose.

WARNING: None of this is information is to be taken lightly, especially if you are an insulin-dependent type-2 diabetic. Restoration of mitochondrial function with proper nutrition, as explained in this book, will subsequently decrease insulin requirements. If insulin is not properly decreased as carbohydrate metabolism is incrementally restored, a hypoglycemic (low blood glucose) episode ***can be life-threatening.***

It is not high glucose that kills acutely; it is dangerously-low glucose that can shut down the brain. Restoring mitochondrial health and careful monitoring of glucose levels go hand-in-hand. Before starting this ten-step program,become your physician. ***Changes in glucose must be closely watched!***

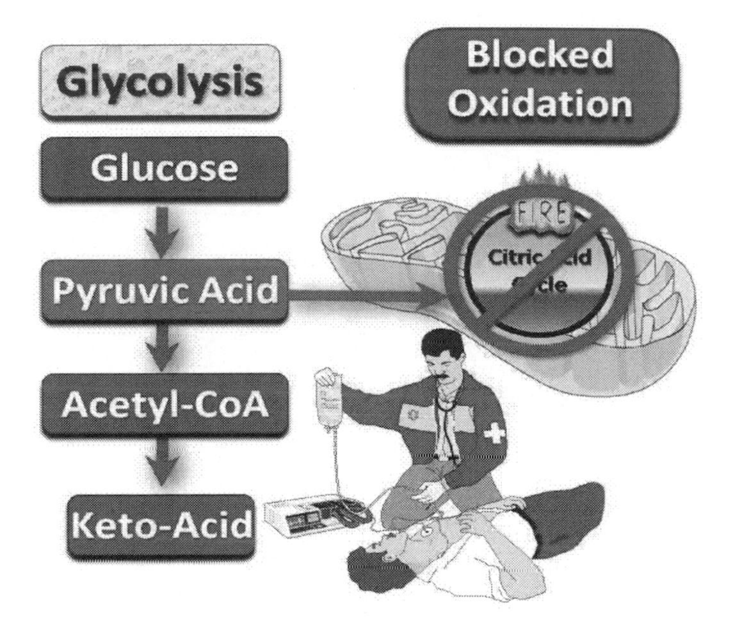

Alternatively, hyperglycemia (high blood glucose) can also lead to emergent hospitalization and even death. This is but another example of the many health hazards from eating nutrient-poor foods that ultimately disable the metabolic machinery of the mighty mitochondria. The metabolic acids that are elevated in emergent cases of hyperglycemia (called *diabetic ketoacidosis*) are keto-acids which can come from incompletely oxidized acetyl-CoA and ***can cause a metabolic coma.***

Bottom Line: Every cell in your body needs ATP to thrive. When your cells make plenty of ATP, you have energy, health and life.

Chapter 27: Big Fat Lies

"The part can never be well unless the whole is well."
-Plato

The key to optimal health is complete oxidation of the carbohydrates you eat. Complete oxidation of a carbohydrate is dependent upon the nutrients within it. The key to eating nutrient-rich carbohydrates is found in eating fresh raw produce – live food not dead food. Yet with all those keys lined up, without healthy mitochondria none of those steps can work very well.

If you tried to start a fire in a broken furnace, all the oxygen, heat and fuel will surely not sustain a fire. If the flue leaks or the metal is fatigued, all your efforts to light a fire with dense dry wood will be wasted. It's no different with your furnaces – the mighty mitochondria where the energy molecules that sustain life are made within membranes.

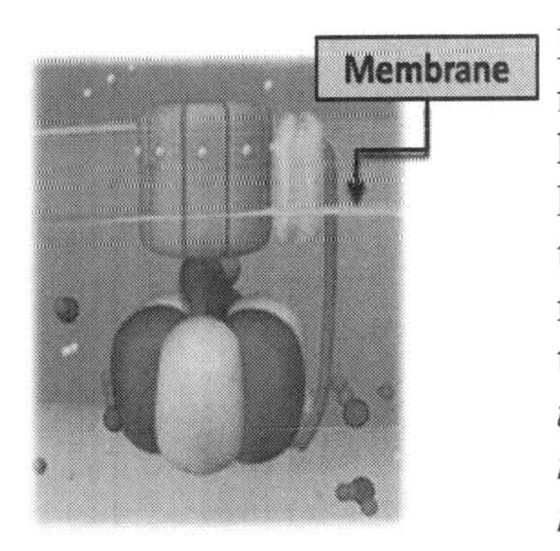

For metabolism to burn brightly, mitochondria must be strong and healthy. In the energy dam, hydrogen from food flows downhill through the inner mitochondrial membrane and spins ATP Synthase to make ATP. ***It is important to note that ATP generation takes place on membranes – and membranes are made mostly of fat.***

Fats are the building blocks of cell membranes and energy production that takes place upon billions of mitochondrial membranes. CWD bacteria invade and consume cholesterol-rich membranes. ***Eating healthy fats, then, is part of the formula for maximizing cellular energy and conquering ALS.***

To prevent fats from breaking down, manufacturers *hydrogenate* vegetable oils, margarine and shortening in order to extend their shelf life. In this process, hydrogen is injected under very high temperatures to make sticky *trans-fats* that stiffen the fat and prevent it from naturally breaking down and becoming rancid.

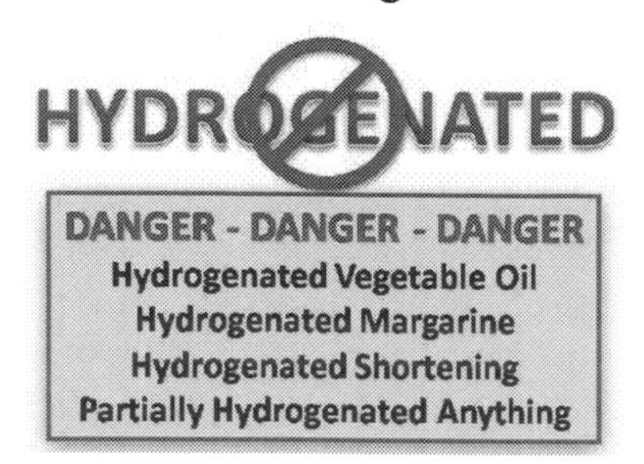

The body inserts these sticky man-made hydrogenated trans-fats into cell membranes. If unnaturally-stiffened margarine and shortening have an endless shelf life, then they likely do inside you. Autoimmune diseases, hardening of the arteries and cancer have increased since the hydrogenation of fats began about a century ago. As a result of incriminating data, some countries have banned all hydrogenated fats from their food supply. Avoid any product with the "H-word" no matter how much good like olive oil is mixed in with the rotten concoction.

Some cooking oils are extracted from vegetable seeds (canola, soybean, vegetable and corn oils) under high temperatures, using petroleum solvents such as hexane that is later boiled off. Some of these oils are also made from "modified" corn and soy which are genetically-modified foods. *Avoid these like a hornets nest.*

Natural fats, on the other hand, naturally break down over time when exposed to light and air. All-natural, solvent-free and cold pressed oils to include olive oil, coconut oil, safflower oil and sesame oil are safe to eat and promote healthy membranes. Included in this list of life-giving fats is butter which should *never* be substituted for man-made lookalikes such as margarine and spreads. Get the fats of life and don't buy the hype.

In the mid-20th century, *saturated* fats such as butter and coconut oil began to receive a lot of bad press – despite that half of the fats in human cell membranes are saturated (with hydrogen) and the other half are unsaturated (contain less hydrogen atoms).

Time and sound science have since shown that two main qualities implicate a fat as a contributor to disease and body fat: 1.) length and 2.) origin (man-made versus natural).

Fats come in three basic sizes: Long, medium and short. Shorter-chain natural fats such as butter and coconut oil are small enough to diffuse into cells without the Carnitine Shuttle. These digestible fats are an instant source of energy, and sometimes this energy burst can be felt within an hour of eating foods cooked with butter or coconut oil. On the other hand, vegetable oils, canola oil and hydrogenated fats such as margarine, spreads and shortening, are long-chain fats that require the Carnitine Shuttle system to be transported into cells for conversion as building blocks for cell membranes or oxidation to acetyl-CoA for making energy. These fats require more work for your cells and are harder to oxidize to make ATP.

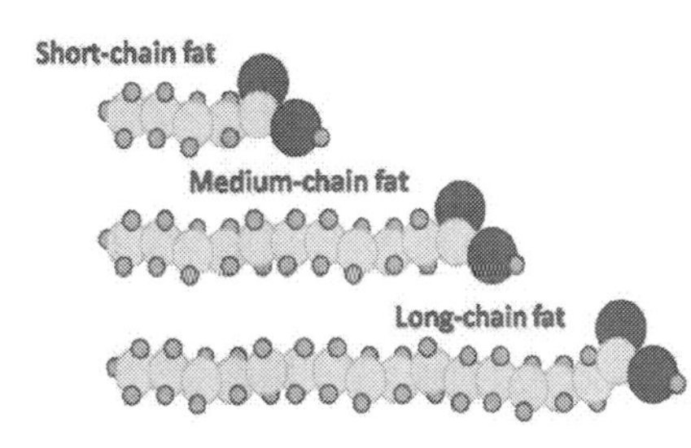

Every cell membrane in your body is made of fats which transport oxygen, chemicals and electrons that are vital for life and energy. When cells are damaged for any reason, hormones called *prostaglandins* are quickly made from cell membrane fats in an effort to respond to the damage.

Prostaglandins regulate important functions such as blood pressure, inflammation and clotting. Over a dozen types of prostaglandins are grouped into three series that trigger various opposing reactions in cells. Series 1 and 2 are made from omega-6 type fats, while Series 3 is made from omega-3 type fats.

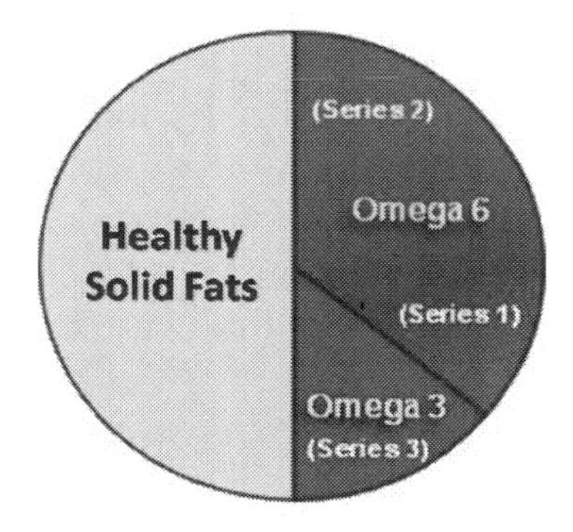

Fifty percent of cell membrane fats are saturated with hydrogen (solid) and the other half are unsaturated (liquid oils). Your diet should therefore reflect the same – half solid fats and half oils, with two-thirds of the oils omega-6 type and one-third omega-3 type. Eating too many omega-6 fats can result in an imbalance of prostaglandins, causing high blood pressure, wheezing, inflammation, pain, clotting, an activated immune system and other serious problems.

Series 1 (Omega 6) & Series 3 (Omega 3)	Series 2 (Omega 6)
Decreases blood pressure	Increases blood pressure
Increases airway dilation	Increases airway constriction
Increases oxygen flow	Decreases oxygen flow
Decreases pain and inflammation	Increases pain and inflammation
Decreases body temperature	Increases body temperature
Suppresses immune system	Activates immune system
Inhibits platelet clotting	Promotes platelet clotting

Most people consume more omega-6 fats then omega-3 fats (more cooking oils than flax oils and fish oil). This is upside down because the electron-rich omega-3 fats are more easily destroyed by industrial oxidizers such as phosphoric acid (in soda) and chlorine (in tap water). This can be corrected by eliminating soda and tap water from the diet and with the old remedy of a daily tablespoon of cod liver oil.

Most people can not tolerate the aftertaste of fish oil (or fish oil supplements). One tablespoons of flaxseed oil mixed in cottage cheese or yoghurt is a tastier substitute. Also, since Series 2 prostaglandins can cause oxidative damage to cell membranes, antioxidants such as vitamin C help ensure cell membranes stay strong and healthy. So, do NOT skip eating lots of raw produce rich in vitamin C and do NOT avoid fats because you need them for healthy cells!

Finally, fat is not what makes fat. It is nutrient-stripped processed carbohydrates that make fat.

Bottom Line: The ATP-making energy process occurs on membranes which are maintained by dietary fat. To make strong and healthy membranes, natural and easily digested fats should be ingested. ***Man-made hydrogenated fats should be avoided at all cost.***

Chapter 28: Dead Food, Dying Cells

"Man cannot live on bread alone."
-Jesus of Nazareth

The cheapest foods are usually the least nutritious foods. One tiny bite can quickly undue a lean physique because food without vitamins cannot completely oxidize. Incompletely oxidized food makes acidic by-products which, over time, lowers the pH of tissues. This sets up an environment for CWD bacteria to invade cells and hide from the immune system while stealing vital cell membranes and myelin sheaths resulting in increasing weakness from nerve degeneration.

Complete oxidation of carbohydrates, on the other hand, is key to a long, healthy life and lean physique.

Nutrient-rich foods arc colorful. Foods rich in vitamin A, for example, are yellow and orange and foods rich in vitamin C are every color of the rainbow – even blue and purple. Processed foods which have been stripped of vitamins are, on the other hand, colorless. To improve sales, colorful cancer-causing dyes are sometimes added.

Why did we start stripping nutrients from our grains in the first place? *Follow the money*. Polished grains such as rice, wheat and barley that have had the vitamin-rich outer husk, bran and germ removed do not spoil. Vitamins B and C quickly oxidize and ruin food. Processing vitamins out of grains therefore gives them more value – long shelf-life value, that is.

If *you*, on the other hand, would like to enjoy an extended life too, then don't eat dead food! Grains are the staple of life; they are used to make bread, pasta, crusts, pastries, cakes, cookies and cereals. All of these delicious foods were once made with hand milled flour (even cereals were freshly milled in the kitchen).

As soon as a grain is cracked and exposed to oxygen, the vitamins immediately begin to oxidize and degrade the grain. When milling was done at home to make fresh unbleached flour or cereal, this nutrient loss was minimized. This is no longer the case with modern food-processing techniques. After all, just look at all the red noses! And even though some B vitamins are added back into flours and cereals (to prevent pellagra), the wrong type of vitamin B3 (nicotinamide) is added. Again, the liver preferentially uses nicotinic acid and not nicotinamide to make NAD.

So, forget all those ***white*** pastries, bagels, croissants, rolls, cookies, cakes and puffed and cracked cereals. Let the dead bury the dead; leave the dead food alone. Dead food can only make dead weight and feed acid-loving microbes.

The same principle applies to sugar. ***White*** sugar has absolutely no nutrients – zilch. It's dead. Bury it. Most brown sugar is the same. It is white sugar with molasses added to darken it.

Avoid processed white foods. White is the color of winter. Choose the vitamin C-rich colorful foods of springtime (green and the all the colors of the rainbow).

If you want to be lean and healthy, then be informed of the nutritional value of every morsel you put into your mouth. Do you want death in your mouth or do you want life? Do you want disease in your gut or do you want health?

If any food you eat is nutritionally wanting, then you, being a sum of your parts, will also be wanting.

And wanting and wanting and wanting, because no matter how much you eat of nutrient-deficient food, you will never be satisfied, your brain simply cannot function without an ample supply of ATP. ***If the food you eat does not contain the nutrients needed to oxidize it completely into ATP, you will forever be burning money on more dead food that never satisfies your hunger and provides health.***

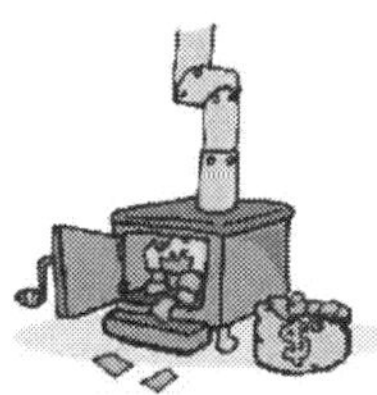

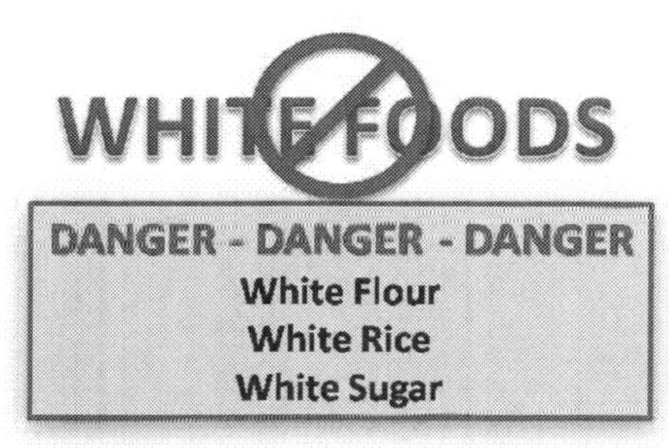

So avoid processed white foods like you would a plague or famine. And if the basic biochemical principals outlined so far in this book haven't convinced you to evict these foods from your cupboards, then try a simple experiment at home. Cook some white rice, throw it on the ground with bird seed and watch. All those bird brains will eat the seed…*but not the cooked white rice*.

Don't be a bird brain. ***Processed food that can sit on a shelf forever is no longer food fit for life.***

Bottom Line: Processed white food is nutrient-dead food with the wrong vitamins mixed back in (if at all). Processed white flour, rice and sugar is not fit for the birds.

Chapter 29: Drug-Induced ALS

"The best doctor uses the least medicines."
-Benjamin Franklin

Not all ALS cases are due to infection with CWD bacteria. ALS can also be induced by man-made chemicals and drugs.

Cholesterol is a steroid molecule resident in cell membranes, nerves and brain tissue. Not unlike collagen, it holds cells, tissues and organs together. It is the building block of vitamin D which is essential to an intact immune system and steroid hormones such as testosterone, progesterone, thyroid hormone, cortisol and aldosterone – all those chemicals that allow our brain to communicate with our organs and make us function normally.

Cholesterol is as essential to life as oxygen. It is so important that CWD bacteria who can not make it will, if given the opportunity, take up residence in human cells and nerves and steal cholesterol to make their own cholesterol-rich membranes. That is why Chlamydia pneumoniae is called an "opportunistic pathogen".

Cholesterol is never "bad". In fact, it is so *good* that cells have two ways to quickly obtain it: 1.) cells take it from the blood as an immediate source when needed to make hormones or grow membranes and 2.) cells make it from scratch.

What is "bad" about cholesterol is its destruction. Fats like cholesterol are electron-rich. It is those electrons that flow through cholesterol that allow nerves to fire and cells to communicate. Ultimately, it is electrons flowing through cholesterol-rich mitochondrial membranes that moves oxidation forward so that ATP is made.

Without electrons flowing through cholesterol-rich membranes, oxidation does not happen. If oxidation does not happen, cells stop “breathing”. When that happens, death follows for cells, organs and the organism. The speed of death depends on how quickly oxidation is arrested.

Strong oxidizing chemicals like chlorine (in tap water), phosphoric acid in soft drinks and tobacco smoke steal electrons from membrane fats like cholesterol. It is *oxidized* (damaged) cholesterol that in turn causes plaques in blood vessels and can cause cardiovascular disease like hardening of the arteries.

Cholesterol is good! OXIDIZED CHOLESTEROL IS BAD! LDL cholesterol is more easily oxidized than HDL cholesterol. That is good for HDL cholesterol, but that does not make HDL cholesterol any more “good” than LDL cholesterol! Cholesterol is so good, and cells need it so much to thrive, that it travels in the blood in dissolved form by binding with proteins. Heavier proteins (High Density Lipoproteins or HDL) protect cholesterol from oxidation more than smaller proteins (Low Density Lipoproteins or LDL). That is bad for LDL cholesterol, but it doesn't make LDL cholesterol “bad”!

Stop buying onto the hype that keeps doctors in the dark selling toxic snake-oil wares like cholesterol-lowering drugs and keeps uninformed people perpetually worried sick and buying more dangerous drugs that make them sicker. If your doctor tells you that you have high “bad” cholesterol, don't try to argue with him or her. *Just run for your life*!

Good life-essential cholesterol is easily oxidized because it is so good at moving electrons and supporting vital life functions like protecting nerves, transmitting signals and making ATP. When cholesterol is destroyed by oxidation on a continual basis, the liver makes and releases it into the blood so that cells in the body have an immediate ready-made supply; blood levels go up.

Because OXIDIZED cholesterol is so bad, ANTI-OXIDANTS help prevent devastating illnesses like heart disease and cancer.

What makes more sense than taking antioxidants is AVOIDING OXIDANTS IN THE FIRST PLACE!!

Want to kill some fish? Put them in a tank of chlorinated tap water and watch them slowly die as their cholesterol-rich scales that provides a water impermeable barrier are slowly oxidized and destroyed by the chlorine. Want to speed up the slow death process? Add some coca cola! Want to slow down or stop the killing spree? Add vitamin C – *a powerful antioxidant.*

Cholesterol is not bad because it carries electrons efficiently and obeys universal chemical laws and is subject to oxidation. CHLORINE IS BAD – IT IS POISON! Fluoride is also an oxidizer like chlorine – it, too, is poison – bad, bad, BAD! Phosphoric acid is BAD – don't drink it! Protect your *good* cholesterol! Without it, you cannot live!

Stop killing yourself. Stop drinking oxidizing acids that destroy cell membranes. Stop listening to and believing in all thc fear mongering that sells sickness.

STOP!! Then, start conquering ALS.

Physicians have not been trained to think as biochemists. Rather, they have been trained to think more likc dispensing pharmacists because it is the pharmaceutical companies that support medical schools through ongoing research and whose always-for-profit study results they buy onto. They consult for drug companies and become brainwashed by hyped up phoney studies (money and true science NEVER mix) and "honoraria" (more money). Upon graduation, doctors are thrown into the clinic setting with one or two lectures on nutrition. Once there, drug reps lurk in clinic hallways with fast answers, free food and loads of study claims to support their drug. With 10 to 15 minutes per patient and a jam packed schedule to juggle every day, doctors fall for fast answers.

Physicians generally don't know enough about how vitamins and minerals tie into human biochemical processes to ask the right questions anyway. They buy the party line of drug reps and prescribe their FDA-approved wares because they believe they will help and not harm. Furthermore, that's all they have. So as to not feel inept, many convince themselves that they have the right answers. Error is perpetuated. As long as everyone sings the same off-tune song from the same page, there is safety in numbers.

Two emotions drive all human behavior: love and fear. One builds up and the other destroys. With a public demand for credibility, doctors inevitably become nurtured by fear which is at the root of bad medicine. To mask the fear, medicine has matured more into the art of practicing magic rather than the art of practicing sound science – replete with magical-sounding names, magical-sounding explanations, magic pills to stop the pain, magical studies to quote…and round and round the spin goes with ever-returning customers rarely getting well. Selling sickness has become big business, despite that some surgeries and antibiotics have lent great credibility to medicine.

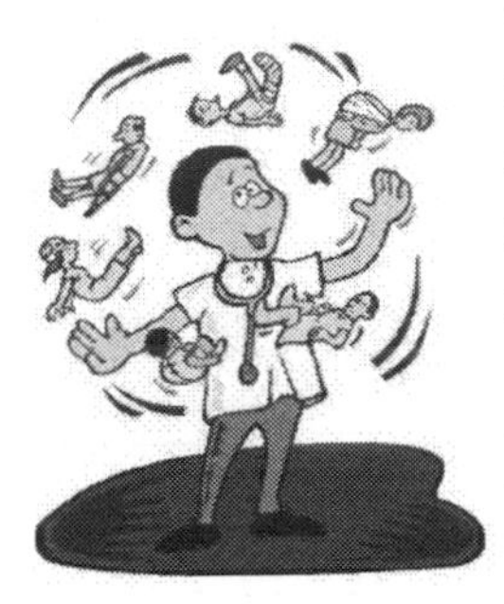

Medical doctors are increasingly duped by pharmaceutical company bogus claims about designer drugs that block symptoms while creating more uncomfortable symptoms that ultimately demand more drugs to block the side effects. Once caught up in the spin, doctors have little time but to use the drugs that everyone else is using (this is called "standard of care") and feed the beast. Healthcare providers, with a desire to help and not harm, boast that their medicine is "evidence-based" – and yet the "evidence" was gathered by companies with an agenda for financial gain. This is not only bad science; it's bad behavior! Sound science and money NEVER mix.

The legalized drug cartel has failed humanity *miserably*. As a single example, consider the number-one selling class of prescription drugs – called "statins" – to lower so-called "bad"

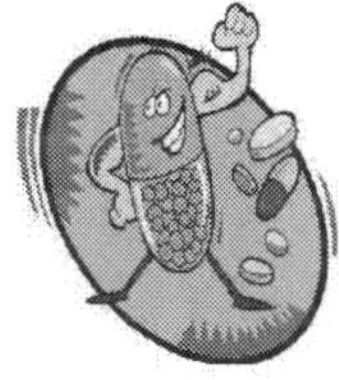

cholesterol. Statin drugs work by blocking a biochemical pathway that all cells use to make various isoprenoids such as cholesterol. Blocking this pathway blocks cells from making isoprenoids needed for replication. If cells can not reproduce, they die. To prevent this, cells respond with a series of life-saving chemical reactions that cause cholesterol to leave the blood and enter into cells. Because blood cholesterol numbers are then lowered, doctors are fooled into thinking they've done some good. It is nothing more than a dangerous chemical “hat trick” (see: “How Statin Drugs Really Lower Cholesterol *And Kill You One Cell at a Time”*).

Blocking cells from making cholesterol can induce ALS. Cholesterol provides structure and a protective barrier to all cell membranes. The central nervous system (brain and spinal cord) makes up 25% of the cholesterol pool. This is because half of the brain matter is cholesterol and nerves are surrounded with a protective wrap called “myelin” that is mostly cholesterol. Myelin is essential for the normal "firing" of nerve signals – not unlike the plastic coating over copper wire that insulates so that electricity flows safely through the wire. Cholesterol is also the building block of steroid hormones such as sex hormones which help make healthy nerves. Predictably, statin users have problems with normal nerve, sexual and muscle function.

A 1999 study demonstrated that *statins kill nerve cells*:

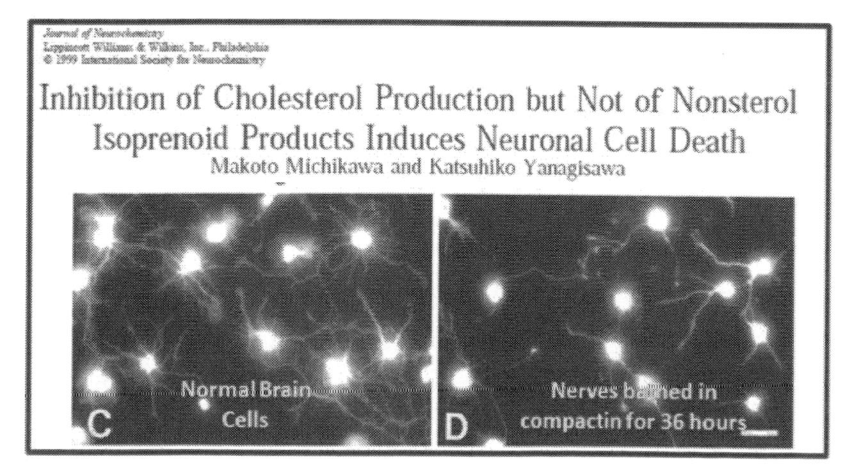
Journal of Neurochemistry
Lippincott Williams & Wilkins, Inc., Philadelphia
© 1999 International Society for Neurochemistry

Inhibition of Cholesterol Production but Not of Nonsterol Isoprenoid Products Induces Neuronal Cell Death

Makoto Michikawa and Katsuhiko Yanagisawa

Experiments on baby rats with cholesterol lowering drugs prove that interruption of cholesterol metabolism alters normal myelination of nerves outside the central nervous system – called "peripheral nerves". These are all the nerves that extend throughout the body from the spinal cord. A normal compact nerve-sheath (left below) degenerates into an abnormally loose arrangement (right below).

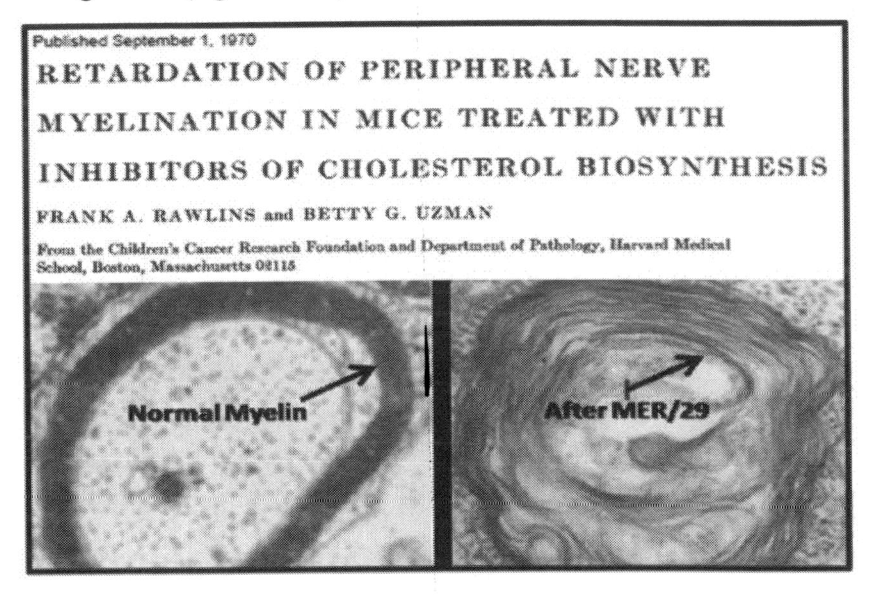
Published September 1, 1970

RETARDATION OF PERIPHERAL NERVE MYELINATION IN MICE TREATED WITH INHIBITORS OF CHOLESTEROL BIOSYNTHESIS

FRANK A. RAWLINS and BETTY G. UZMAN

From the Children's Cancer Research Foundation and Department of Pathology, Harvard Medical School, Boston, Massachusetts 02115

Physicians in Denmark found that people taking statins were more likely to develop peripheral neuropathy – characterized by weakness, tingling and pain in the hands and feet and difficulty walking – all symptoms of drug-induced ALS. Taking statins for two or more years raised the risk of nerve damage by 26 percent:

Statins and risk of polyneuropathy

NEUROLOGY 2002;58:1333–1337

A case-control study

D. Gaist, MD, PhD; U. Jeppesen, MD, PhD; M. Andersen, MD, PhD; L.A. García Rodríguez, MD, MSc; J. Hallas, MD, PhD; and S.H. Sindrup, MD, PhD

For patients treated with statins for 2 or more years the odds ration of definite idiopathic polyneuropathy was 26.4 (7.8 to 45.4). *Conclusions:* Long-term exposure to statins may substantially increase the risk of polyneuropathy.

The Danish study (published in 2002) was not the first to implicate statins in the development of nerve problems with ALS like symptoms. While developing the first statin in the 1980's, Merck had already discovered the neurotoxic multiple scarring (ALS) effects of lovastatin in their experimental dogs – but did not publish this finding until 1988 – one year after the drug was FDA approved. Photo "B" below is a sample of a dog's brain after 12 days of ingesting lovastatin:

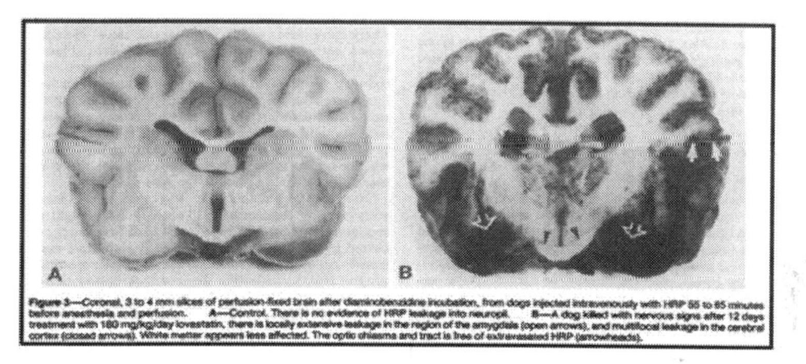

Figure 3—Coronal, 3 to 4 mm slices of perfusion-fixed brain after diaminobenzidine incubation, from dogs injected intravenously with HRP 55 to 65 minutes before anesthesia and perfusion. A—Control. There is no evidence of HRP leakage into neuropil. B—A dog killed with nervous signs after 12 days treatment with 180 mg/kg/day lovastatin, there is locally extensive leakage in the region of the amygdala (open arrows), and multifocal leakage in the cerebral cortex (closed arrows). White matter appears less affected. The optic chiasma and tract is free of extravasated HRP (arrowheads).

Statins block a biochemical pathway used by cells to make various isoprenoids (five-carbon fatty electron-rich molecules). Cholesterol is but one of many of these vital-to-life isoprenoids. CoQ10 is another.

CoQ10 is just as essential as oxygen and NAD for oxidative metabolism to occur. The hydrogen energy-dam that ultimately makes ATP is the result of work performed within an entire complex of proteins embedded in the inner mitochondrial membrane. Some of these proteins are mobile and others are not. CoQ10 is one of two *mobile* proteins in this complex. Without CoQ10, cells can not make ATP very well – *if at all.*

Carbohydrates are metabolized into hydrogen atoms which are delivered to the ATP-making complex by NAD. A hydrogen atom is comprised of one electron and one proton. When NAD delivers hydrogen atoms to the first protein complex, the electron and proton are separated, and hydrogen *protons* are pumped across the membrane into the "hydrogen or proton energy dam" that in turn spins ATP Synthase to make ATP.

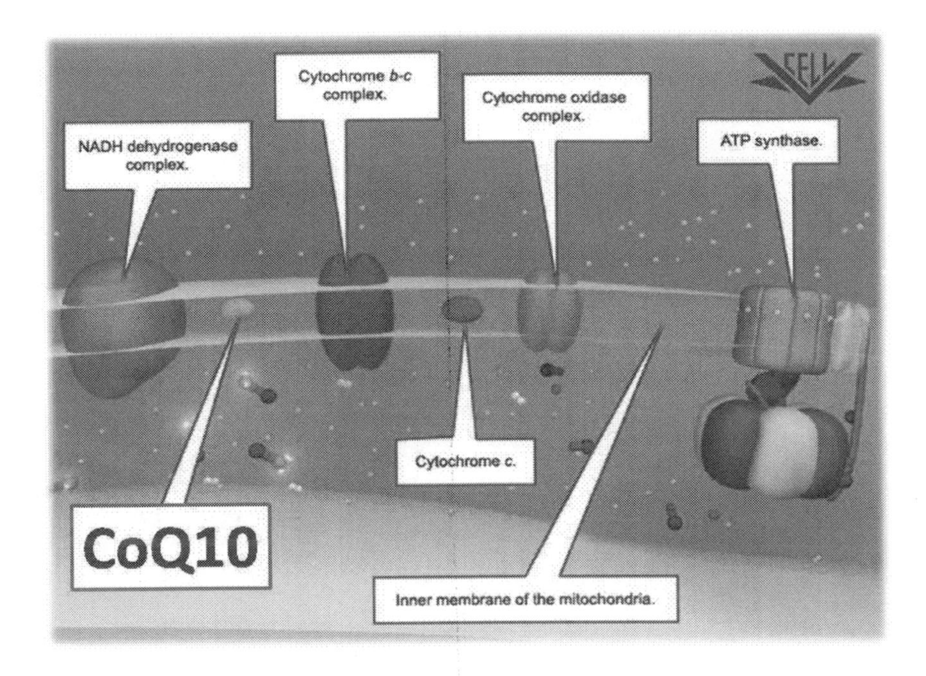

The electrons, in turn, are transported to the next protein molecule by CoQ10 – hence giving rise to the term "electron transport chain" for this final stage of oxidation. Without this process of electrons being propelled forward by CoQ10, the whole process can only be slowed down or completely stopped.

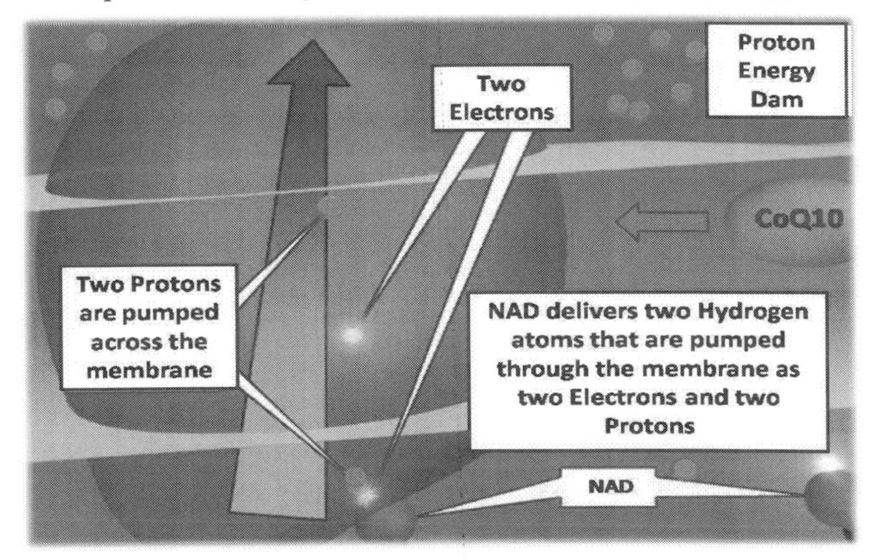

Blocking CoQ10 therefore blocks the entire ATP-making machinery and shuts down your life generating batteries. This results in a whole host of ill effects: fatigue, difficulty thinking, painful muscles, muscle cell destruction, demyelination of nerves and polyneuropathy – all symptoms of ALS. Do doctors know these small but vital details? No, they generally do not! If these risks are not disclosed to them, they cannot pass it on to their patients.

But if the doctor thinks it's good for you, it must be good, right?

Wrong. Dead wrong. Part of conquering ALS is avoiding dangerous drugs and chemicals that can damage your nerves.

Cholesterol is good. It is not a good idea to try to block cells from making it. Doing so is not only dangerous in itself, it also blocks cells from making ATP which is the energy molecule of life.

Without sufficient ATP, a cell cannot function normally.

Bottom Line: Treating disease by blocking or circumventing normal biochemical processes with drugs does not restore health because health restoration is not part of the design. Furthermore, some drugs like statins induce debilitating diseases with ALS-like symptoms. This is called drug-induced ALS.

Chapter 30: Second Steps

"Time heals all wounds."
-Anonymous

The protective myelin wrap around nerves is essential for the normal "firing" of nerve signals – like plastic coating insulates copper wire so that electricity flows safely. Important nutrients that help make glial cells grow and replicate include: cholesterol, sex hormones, essential fatty acids, lecithin, choline, inositol, B vitamins (especially B12) and minerals.

The foods that are richest in these nutrients are: eggs, eggs, eggs! Fried, scrambled, poached or pickled, eat as many as you want or as many as you can. Eggs will NOT increase your cholesterol! (Smoking or drinking oxidizing fluids will – so if you smoke, try to cut back or quit.) If you are middle-aged and have lost your libido, it may return as you eat plenty of eggs. That is because progesterone and testosterone are made from cholesterol.

If you don't have your own backyard chickens, it's well worth the effort to drive to a country homestead that sells fresh eggs from free range chickens. These (normal) eggs typically have a beautiful dark yellow or orange yolk – full of vitamins from the greens that free-range chickens enjoy and passed on to you.

The sex hormones progesterone and testosterone are important for nerve health and re-myelination. Pregnenolone is a natural supplement that is the precursor molecule for cells to make progesterone and testosterone; it is suitable for both men and women. Some people report more energy and ability to focus with pregnenolone, so as a supplement it is taken in the morning. In addition to pregnenolone, natural plant-derived progesterone and estrogen creams for women and testosterone cream for men will support the re-myelination process. These are readily available in most vitamin and health food stores. I've found the best selection and prices on-line at Iherb.com.

After eggs, pregnenolone and hormone cream supplements every morning, eat raw nuts and seeds throughout the day. These are rich in B vitamins and minerals. Once or twice a day ingest two tablespoons of flax oil mixed in cottage cheese or yoghurt (as explained in Part Three to follow).

In Part Three, the ten-step ALS diet provides a wide array of foods and drinks that support oxidative metabolism and maximum ATP production. For one to three months (or as long as you continue to see notable improvements), however, I recommend a food and supplement regimen that diverts from the variety of the ALS diet to instead focus on foods and supplements that will support nerve re-myelination (First Steps and Second Steps).

If you have been following the first steps in this book, then you have already begun to slowly change your body water to a lightly basic pH by doing the following:

FIRST STEPS

DRINK:

Non chlorinated well-mineralized water (never distilled water)
Juice from 12 freshly-squeezed apples (strain the foam)

(Option: Core and peel the apples before juicing and use the pulp to make apple sauce cooked in water, stevia and cinnamon.)

SUPPLEMENTAL MINERALS:

Calcium citrate capsules (night)
Magnesium malate capsules (morning)
Alka-Selzer (at least twice daily); salt on food
Cell Food – as directed

After a minimum of two weeks of the First Steps protocol, proceed to the Second Steps:

SECOND STEPS

SUPPLEMENTAL VITAMINS

Multi-vitamin gel caps/NAD lozenges/B12 spray as directed

SUPPLEMENTAL PROBIOTICS (Anti-toxin effectors):

Probiotics – Acidophilus and Bifidobacterium – as directed.
MOS – Mannan Oligosaccharides – as directed.

SUPPLEMENTAL HORMONES (if over 50, have been taking statins and/or have decreased libido):

Men and women: Pregnenolone 50 mg (in morning, as directed)
Women: Progesterone cream (as directed)
Men: Male performance gel (as directed)

BREAKFAST:

3-8 egg omelette cooked in safflower oil. Filler choices: mushroom, onion, tomato, spinach, peppers (any kind), goat cheese, broccoli, asparagus. Season with iodized salt and as desired. Top with raw diced sweet onion (as much as you can eat) and parmesan. Apple juice. Optional: salsa topping.

SNACK:

Raw nuts mixed with raw sunflower and pumpkin seeds (raisins, dates and dried apples if desired); raw fruit/vegetables/avocados.

Yogurt with live active cultures (Acidophilus and Bifidobacterium).

Dice 4 tomatoes and 2 sweet onions into a bowl blended with 2-4 packets of stevia. Add apple cider or balsamic vinegar, salt, parmesan and spices to taste. Alternative: Homemade tomato soup topped with raw diced sweet onion. Eat throughout the day.

LUNCH/DINNER:

Flax fiesta (page 160) with 2-4 tablespoons of flax oil. If you don't like cottage cheese, mix flax oil in yogurt (labeled with "active live culture") or unsweetened apple sauce with stevia and cinnamon to taste. Apple juice.

Meals of choice from recipes in Part Three; fresh deep sea fish (avoid farm raised tilapia, basa or catfish) is always preferable for meat. Apple juice.

These are samples of the above listed supplements that I have found to be the best quality at discount prices (from Iherb.com). Coupon code "YEN890" is an additional 5% first order discount.

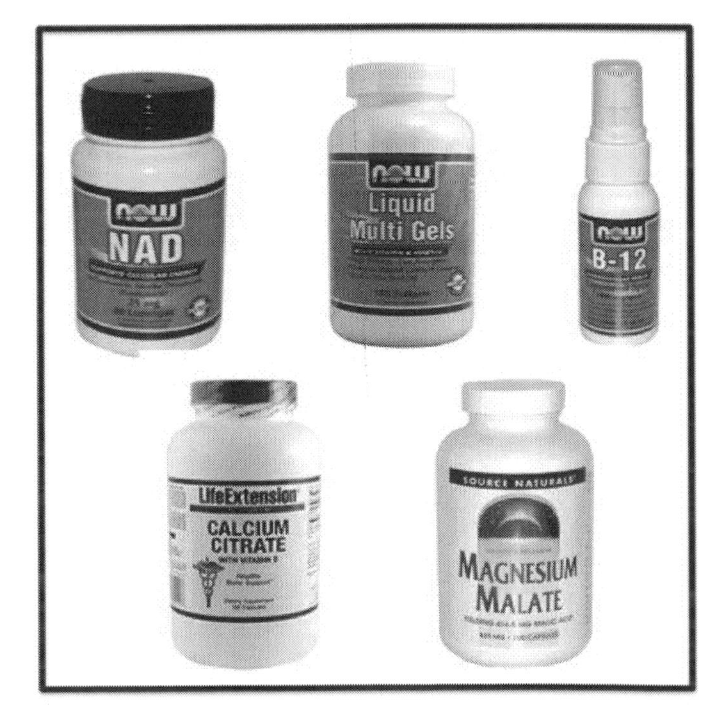

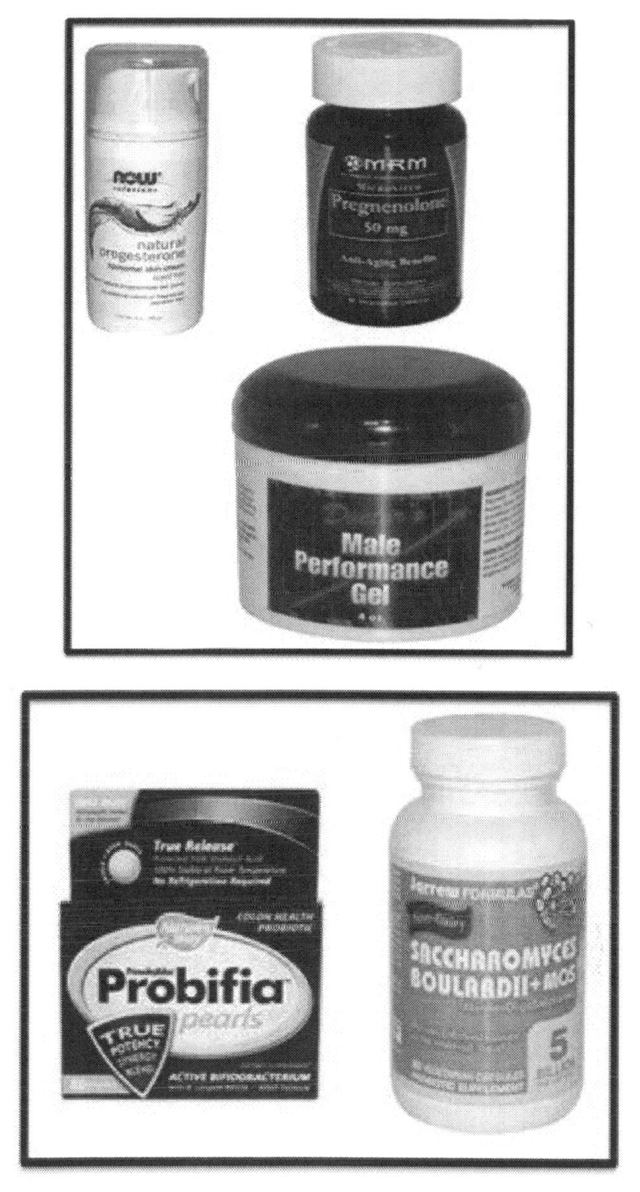

Remember, while healing you may have one or more healing crises (also called a "Herxheimer reaction"). As your body water begins to alkalinize and anaerobic microbes die off, you may experience *extreme* fatigue, muscle aches, fever and other flu-like symptoms for days to weeks. These are all signs that the immune system is hard at work cleaning up the "debris". Be encouraged.

The early healing phase can be very uncomfortable so make slow changes to your body chemistry! If this happens, you may want to stop taking some or all of the supplements and restart them one at a time to find out what is causing the discomfort.

NAD, B-12, magnesium malate and pregnenolone are all widely reported to increase energy without jittery, heart-stimulating side effects. Take these in the morning. Calcium has a calming effect and should be taken at night. The liquid multi gels energize some people and others become fatigued; find out what works for you. Whether taken at morning or night, all of the pill form supplements should be taken with food.

When your strength, energy and balance are noticeably improving, enjoy the variety of nutritious foods (real food!) from the powerful ATP-producing and healthy nerve-firing ALS diet to follow in Part Three.

Bottom Line: Important foods for conquering ALS are eggs, apples (and home made apple juice), raw onion, raw tomatoes, raw nuts, raw seeds, yogurt (with live active cultures) and flax oil. Be prepared to feel worse before you feel better.

PART THREE: THE ALS DIET

Step 1: Clean up Your Swimming Pool

This is what a picture of $100-worth of health restoring food looks like. Eating more of these foods will help guarantee you long life, health and vitality.

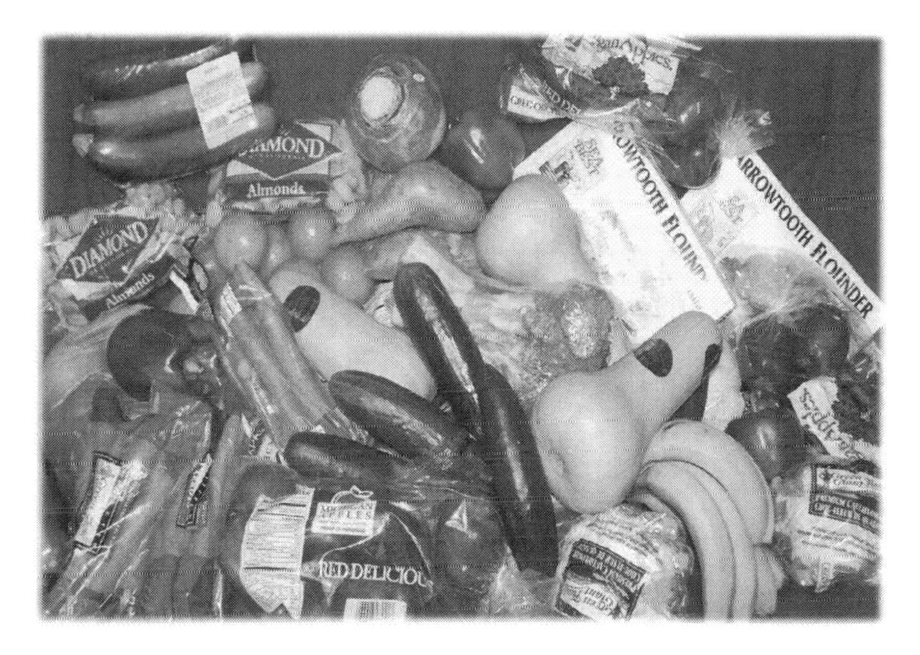

With the exception of the raw almonds, all of these wholesome foods are found around the *outside walls* of a grocery store and *not in the aisles*. With rare exception, if you want to lose excess fat and/or restore lost health, avoid shopping in the aisles. There you will find mostly refined food that makes acid and fat.

Included in the above photo are apples, oranges, tangerines, grapefruit, bananas, raw almonds, cauliflower, broccoli, yams, rutabaga, various types of squash, cucumber, bell pepper, onions and carrots. Buried under that heap of vitamin C rich foods are two more bags of apples for a total of five three-pound bags of apples for ten days of fat-burning energy-packed food. *That* is real food.

You are 50-70 percent water, and the mighty ATP-making mitochondria are bathed in this water. Since a basic pH is required for the energy-making process to operate well, the first step to take on your journey to health restoration and/or a lean body is to clean up your swimming pool. This requires restoring and maintaining your body water at a pH that promotes cellular oxidation.

Step One: Clean up your swimming pool.

Juice	**Fresh-squeezed Citrus, apple and carrot**
Water	**Fluoride-free** ***NOT DISTILLED!***
Green/Herbal Tea	**As much as you like!**

If you drink soda pop then STOP! Optimum oxidation requires a basic water pH of 7.4. This allows NAD to deliver hydrogen atoms into the hydrogen energy dam and create an acidic, low-pH environment *above* the dam where a *difference* in the concentration of hydrogen atoms (pH difference) above and below the dam creates a gradient for hydrogen to flow "downhill" through ATP Synthase and make ATP.

Excess acid that kidneys can't filter out inevitably weakens the pH difference across the mitochondrial dam. Since it is a difference in the potential of hydrogen atoms that drives the ATP energy making process, an excess of hydrogen from dietary acids compromises the hydrogen (pH) differential across the dam.

A compromised dam means low ATP which means low energy; a broken dam means no energy. YOU CAN NOT CONQUER ALS AND DRINK SODA – PERIOD.

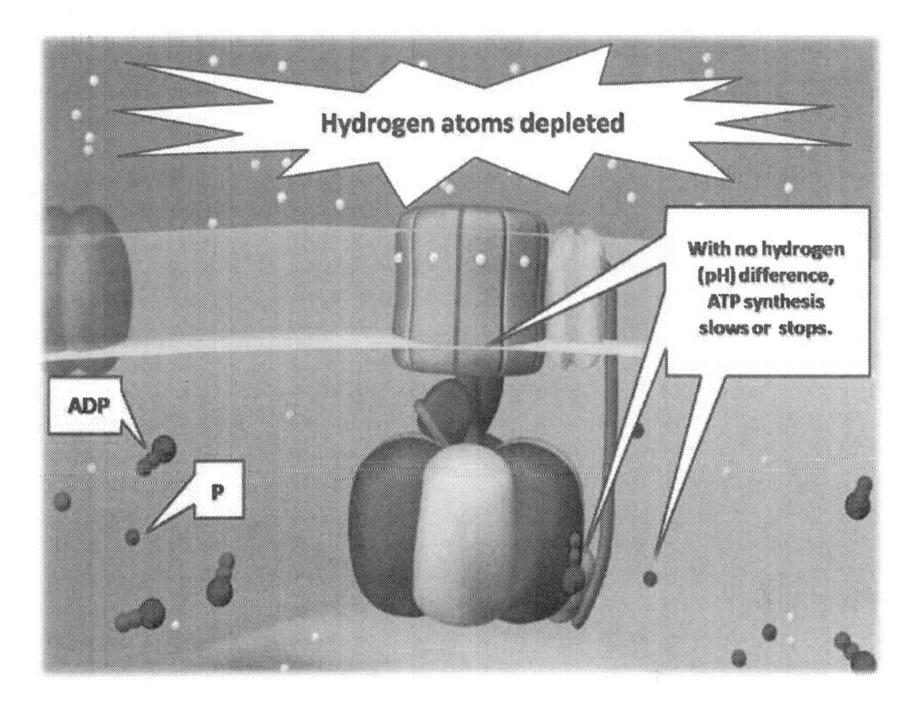

Oxygen is required for oxidation to work efficiently. The lower the pH of a water, the less oxygen is present. If you smoke, cut back or quit; this decreases cellular oxygen and hinders oxidation (that's why smokers huff and puff)!

When cellular oxidation is hindered, glycolysis prevails. Where glycolysis prevails, so do pathogenic microbes that make energy by glycolysis. And since the by-products of glycolysis include fat and acid, drinking diet soda is one of the surest ways to get sick AND fat.

Fat and chronic disease are both a four-letter word: ACID. You also will need to stop drinking all alcoholic drinks, including wine, until your weight and/or health return to normal. This, too, is not negotiable. Vitamins B and C which are key nutrients in the energy-making process are easily destroyed by alcohol.

If you are addicted to coffee try to cut back as much as possible, and preferably completely, until you have reached your optimum weight and health. Coffee, which does contain vitamin B3 as nicotinic acid, has certain acids which, unlike malic acid in apples and citric acid in citrus fruits, does *not* directly fuel the citric acid cycle.

With the exception of non-distilled bottled spring water or seltzer water, eliminate all man-made drinks. Juices, even if found in the cooler section rather than the center aisles, are pasteurized or flash-pasteurized – hence most if not all of the vitamins are destroyed. ***Eliminate all sports' drinks, sodas (except seltzer), flavored waters, chlorinated tap water or powdered drink mixes.***

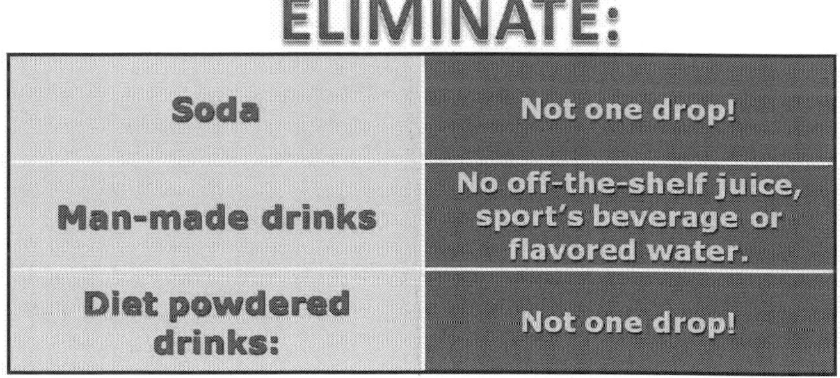
ELIMINATE:

Soda	Not one drop!
Man-made drinks	No off-the-shelf juice, sport's beverage or flavored water.
Diet powdered drinks:	Not one drop!

There is no need for trendy or expensive detoxification programs or supplements; restoring your body to its naturally basic pH, while eliminating old acid-forming foods and drinks, will detoxify your body, naturally, with time. Be patient. Remember, a basic pH is nature's ultimate antibiotic for eliminating acid-loving, disease-causing microbes.

The first food to prepare at the start of the day is a two day supply of freshly-squeezed juice. Some of the least expensive juicers work the best at extracting the most juice from fruit (such as the $50 black plastic GE juicer from Wal Mart).

Fat-Melting Energy-Packed Juice

3-pounds of apples
3 pink peeled grapefruit
3 peeled oranges

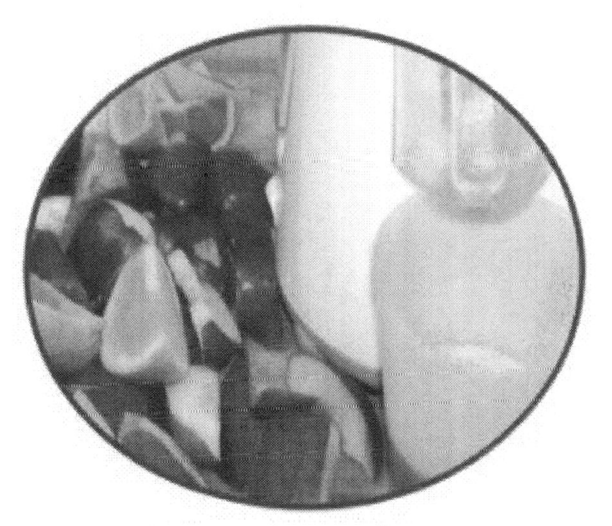

6 carrots (optional)
1-pound of grapes (optional)

Slice apples to fit in juicer.
Cut grapefruit and oranges in quarters. Remove rinds.
Wash carrots and slice lengthwise as needed to fit in juicer.

You may need to open the juicer lid occasionally to remove pulp and peels that do not evacuate into the waste bin. Because vitamin C is degraded as soon as it is exposed to oxygen, this juice should be freshly made every other day. One 16-ounce glass of this fresh apple-citrus-carrot juice is packed with so much vitamin C and nutrients for fueling the citric acid cycle (malic acid, citric acid, calcium and magnesium) that you will find this drink not only satisfies morning hunger, but you should have more energy to last throughout the day.

Freshly made juice will elevate blood sugar but not for long. If you have type 2 diabetes, check your glucose before, one hour after and four hours after drinking this juice. You will likely find that despite an initial glucose spike one hour after drinking the juice your over glucose levels trend will downward. Keep records, inform your physician and ensure your diabetes medications are adjusted accordingly.

To make use of the pulp from making juice, peel and juice carrots first. Remove the carrot pulp and cook in water, salt and seasons to taste to make carrot soup (topped with raw diced onion and parmesan). Clean the hopper; juice apples with peels and cores removed. Remove the apple pulp and cook in water, stevia and cinnamon to taste to make apple sauce. Last, juice the citrus and discard or compost the citrus pulp.

Drink as much fresh juice as you want as often as you want; the more, the better. The more you drink, the more carnitine will be made to heal cells, burn stored fat and acids and release more energy. This powerful health restoring formula is all in keeping with the father of medicine's advice, using proven biochemical principals.

There is no carbohydrate combination like apples and citrus fruit that directly fuels the citric acid cycle and, in so doing, pushes oxidation to the full "on" mode to burn up painful dietary acids that have been storing up in muscles and organs.

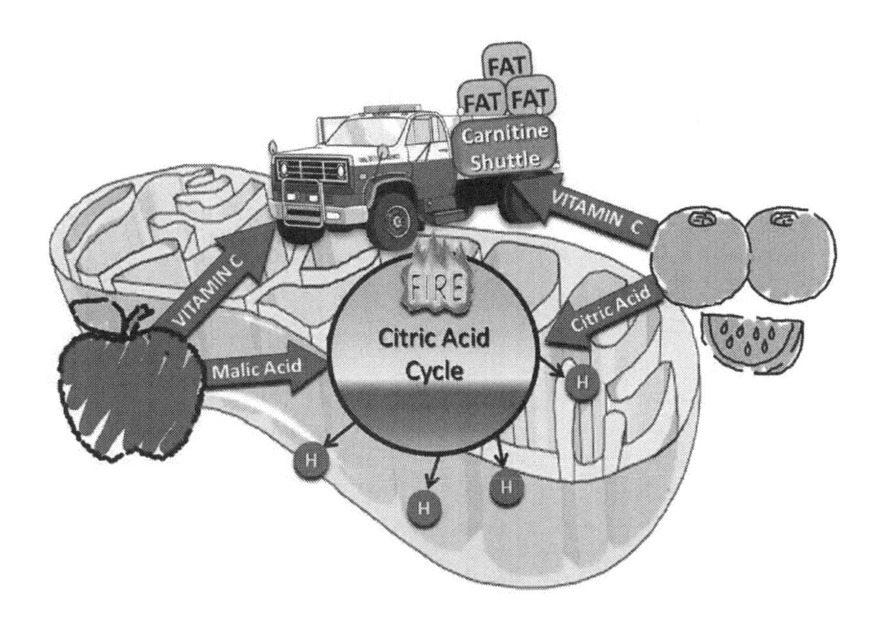

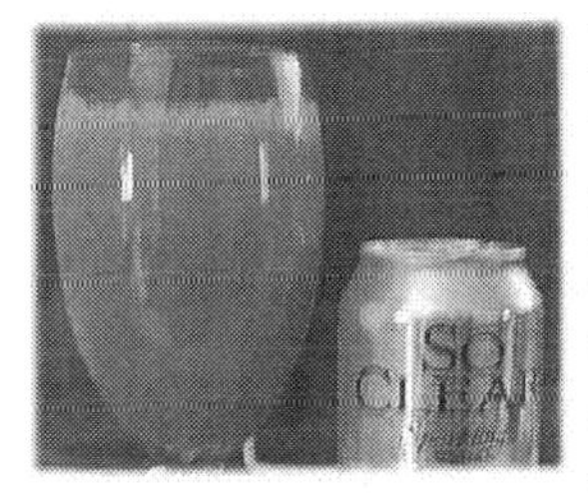

If you miss soft drinks, then add seltzer water ("sparkling water") to your freshly made juice with a 50/50 mix. Seltzer water has a neutral pH and is acid-free. Now you can enjoy a healthy and delicious soda concoction as you drink up and clean up your pool!

"Those who think they have no time for healthy eating will sooner or later have to find time for illness."
-Edward Stanley

Step 2: Eat C-Food

Because vitamin C makes collagen which makes cells, tissues and organs strong, vitamin C-rich foods are key to conquering ALS. The key is to minimize over-heating and over-chilling so as to preserve the temperature sensitive vitamin.

Step Two: Eat C-Food.

Squash	**Summer, zucchini, butternut, acorn and spaghetti squash Cucumber**
Onions & Tomatoes	***Powerful foods!***
Other	**Cabbage, broccoli, cauliflower, peppers, green beans, greens, spinach and mushrooms**

One of the best sources of vitamin C is squash which should be a frequent addition to any eat-more-not-less meal (this includes cucumber which is in the squash family). Squash is so nutrient-packed and therefore appetite-suppressing that just half of a butternut squash makes a satisfying meal. Cut butternut and acorn squash lengthwise in half, scoop out the seeds and cook them upside-down and covered in a microwave for 8 minutes. Cool and let them soften for an additional five minutes before further cooking. While microwave-heating destroys some vitamins, I've found that cooked butternut and acorn squash still promote weight loss. Season them to taste with butter, garlic powder, salt and pepper.

This recipe, which will last for days when refrigerated, makes a delicious raw vegetable side dish that's packed with nutrients:

C-MORE VEGGIES

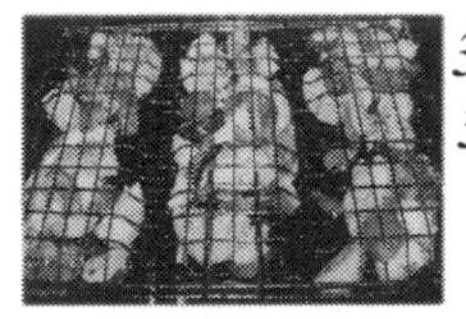

3 zucchini and 3 yellow squash
3 tomatoes, 2 onions, 1 pepper
½ cup balsamic vinegar
½ cup olive oil
Parmesan cheese
Seasonings

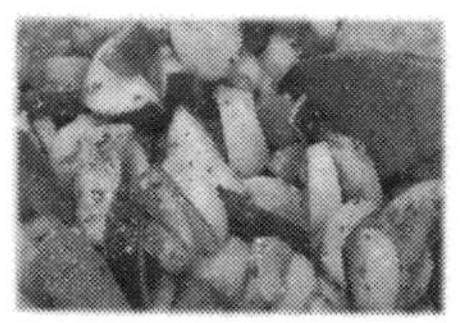

Cut the above vegetables into bite-size pieces and set aside. Whisk together the vinegar and oil and garnish with parmesan cheese and seasonings (season-salt, pepper, garlic and herbs). Blend the oil-vinegar-seasonings mixture into the vegetables. Serve raw or quickly-seared on a grill.

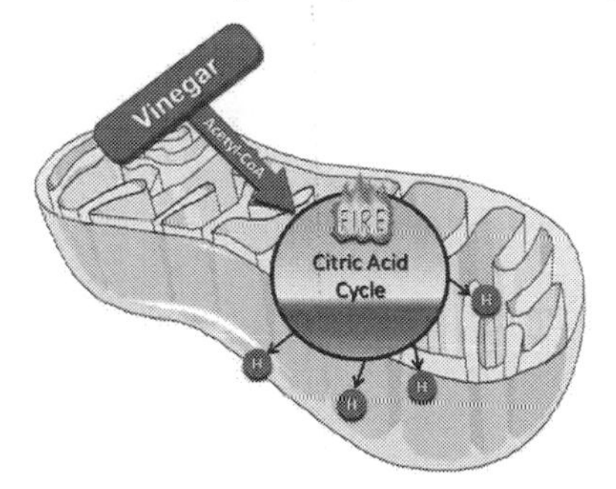

The longer these vegetables marinate in the vinegar-based mixture, the better they will taste – even raw! Vinegar is acetic acid which is readily converted into acetyl-CoA which feeds the citric acid cycle. Apple cider vinegar, which also contains malic acid from apples, gives the citric acid an extra ATP-packing punch. I've chosen the subtle flavor of balsamic vinegar, however, for the above recipe.

Spaghetti squash makes a delightful substitute for pasta. Because pasta is made from processed grains, it's an acid-making carbohydrate (even "whole wheat" pasta is stripped of nutrition and is mostly white flour). Spaghetti squash cut in half, with seeds removed and cooked in the microwave, will

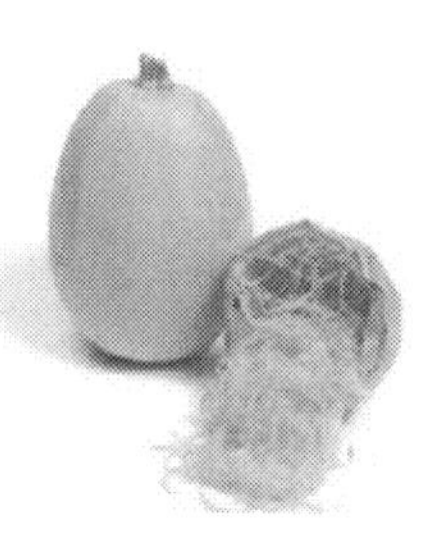

scrape from the rind like spaghetti. Top this with your favorite tomato sauce or chili and top with raw diced sweet onion. Eat as much as you want.

Tomatoes and onions are some of the most nutritious carbs. Four foods that have been found to significantly reduced heart disease (by more than 25%) are 1.) tomatoes, 2.) onions, 3.) apples and 4.) broccoli. The key ingredient in these four foods is vitamin C which makes collagen and keeps blood vessels healthy and strong. Raw or cooked, the more you eat of these while avoiding nutrient-poor processed foods, the more vitamin C will convert to carnitine and collagen and the more strong tissues you will gain. Vitamin C also makes collagen that makes skin look and feel firm. Nails that used to be weak and brittle will become noticeably stronger and fungus-free.

Next in line to fresh apple-citrus juice, the ALS diet "top ten" list of C-foods are:

Tomatoes
Onions
Squash and cucumber
Cabbage
Cauliflower
Broccoli
Bean Sprouts
Carrots
Mushrooms
Greens: Kale, mustard and spinach

Try to add diced raw sweet onion on top of every possible cooked food and/or garnish a plate with raw sliced tomatoes.

Here are a variety of ways to prepare these ten C-foods (tomatoes and onions are a frequent addition as these two carbohydrates are the top two of these top ten foods):

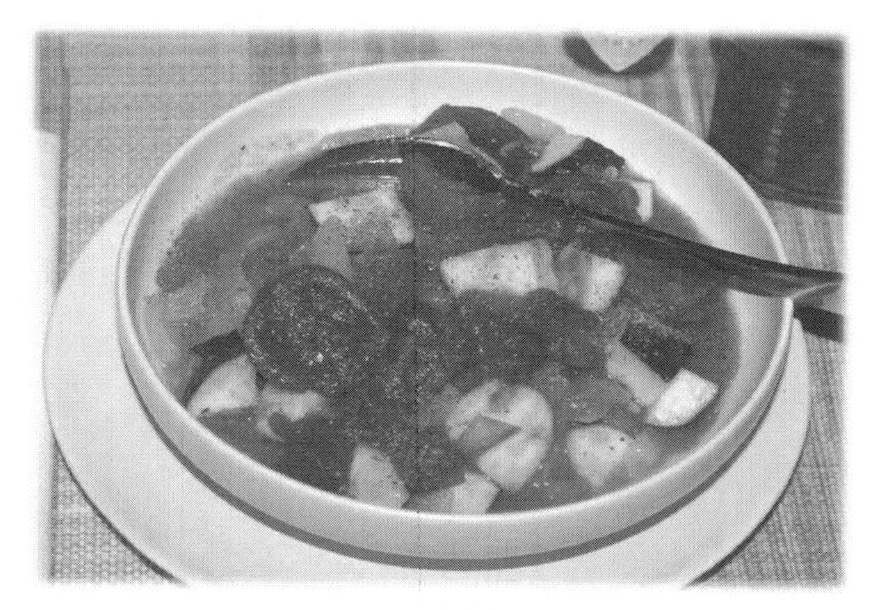

GET-UP-AND-GO STEW

4 sweet onions
4 tomatoes
4 zucchini
28-ounce can crushed tomatoes
Raw sugar
Seasonings
Parmesan cheese/Diced raw sweet onion

Dice onions and sauté in 2 tablespoons coconut, olive or sesame seed oil.
Season to taste (season salt, pepper, garlic and curry).
Add sliced tomatoes and sauté 5 minutes.
Add canned tomatoes and 2 tablespoons of raw sugar.
Heat to a low boil.
Add sliced zucchini and cook for 3 minutes.
Garnish with parmesan cheese and diced raw sweet onion.

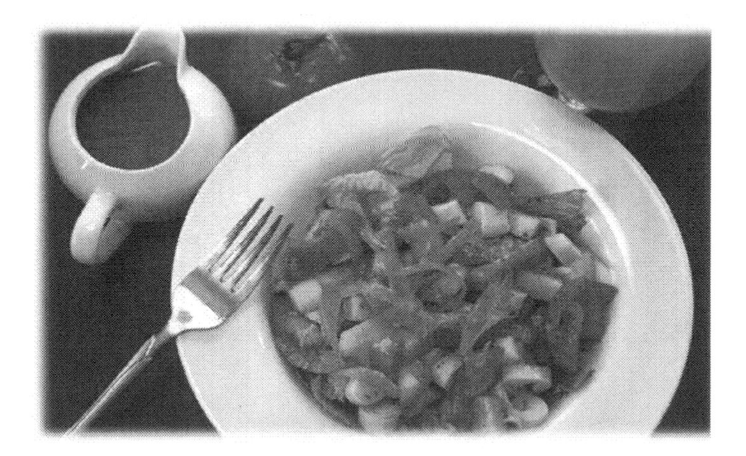

PALM GARDEN SALAD

1 can hearts-of-palm
1 cucumber, 1 tomato, 1 carrot
Lettuce

Slice hearts-of-palm, cucumber and tomato.
Serve on a bed of lettuce and top with grated carrot.
Garnish with almond-ginger vinaigrette dressing.

Almond-Ginger Vinaigrette

1 teaspoon almond butter
1 teaspoon grated ginger root
¾ cup olive oil
3 tablespoons apple cider vinegar
1 teaspoon brown rice miso
1 tablespoon sesame tahini
2 tablespoons raw honey
1 crushed garlic clove
¼ teaspoon basil
¼ teaspoon sea salt

Mix above ingredients in blender.

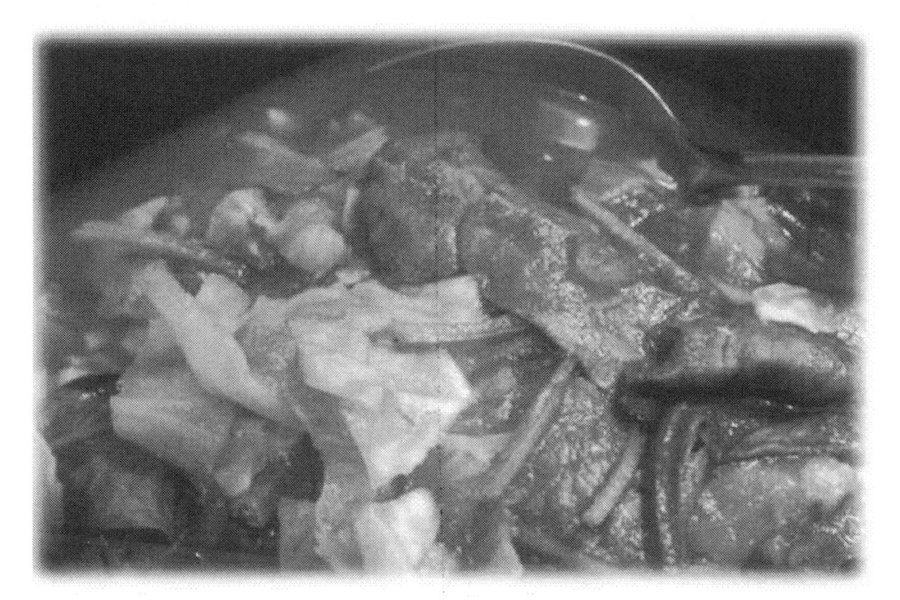

CABBAGE CABOODLE

1 head of cabbage
1 bag of fresh spinach
Two 28-ounce cans crushed tomatoes
Raw sugar
Seasonings
Parmesan cheese/Diced raw sweet onion.

Bring two cans of stewed tomatoes to low boil.
Season tomatoes to taste (stevia, salt, pepper, herbs).
Fold in diced cabbage and cook for 5 minutes.
Turn off heat and fold in spinach.
Garnish with parmesan cheese and diced raw sweet onion.

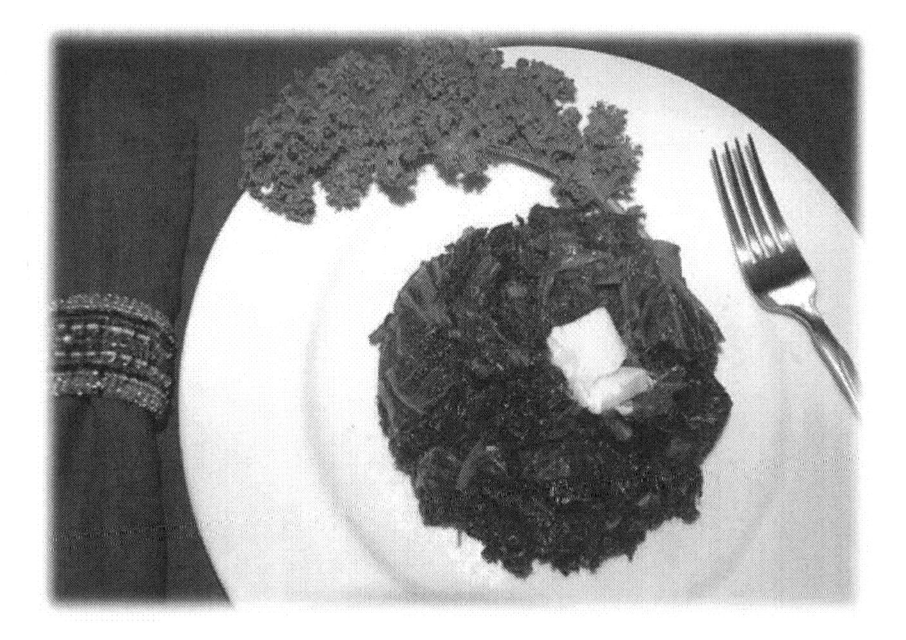

ENVIOUS GREENS

One bunch each of mustard and kale greens
Apple cider vinegar
Olive oil
Stevia
Butter, sea salt and pepper

Wash greens and remove thick stems.
Add one inch of water and greens to pot.
Boil then cook on low-medium heat until cooked (about one hour).
Drain water and chop greens.
Mix 1-2 tablespoons each of vinegar, oil and sugar to taste.
Add butter, sea salt and pepper to taste.

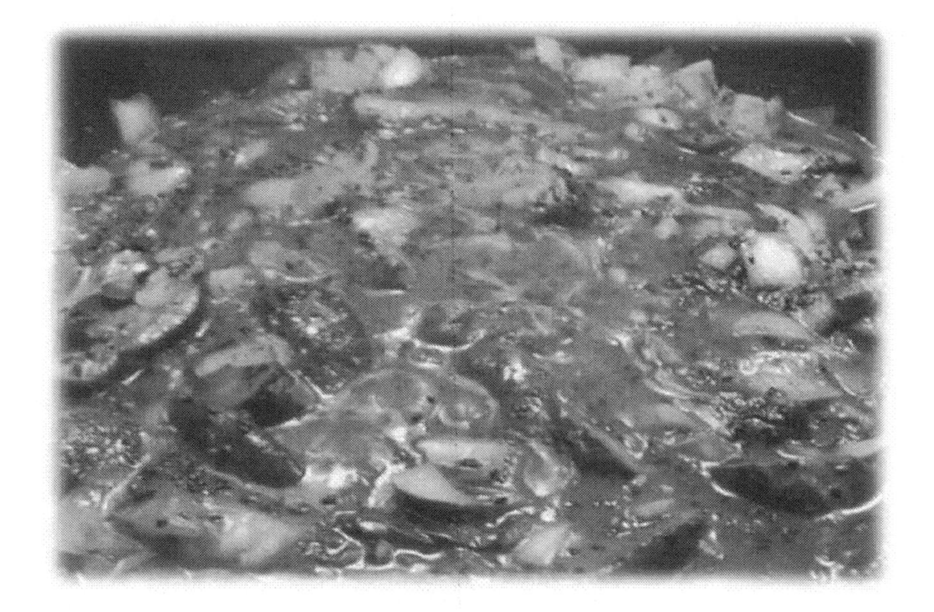

SHITAKE FEST

10 shitake mushrooms
2 sweet onions
2 tomatoes
4 tablespoons sesame seeds (black or white)
28-ounce can crushed tomatoes
Seasonings
Parmesan cheese/Diced raw sweet onion

Sauté sesame seeds, until brown, in 2 tablespoons of coconut, olive or sesame oil.
Remove seeds from pan.
Sauté sliced onions in 2 tablespoons of coconut, olive or sesame oil for 5 minutes.
Stir in sliced raw tomatoes and cook for 3 minutes.
Add stewed tomatoes, cooked sesame seed and mushrooms.
Cook 5 more minutes and season to taste.
Garnish with parmesan cheese and/or diced raw sweet onion.
Optional: Fold in raw spinach leaves.

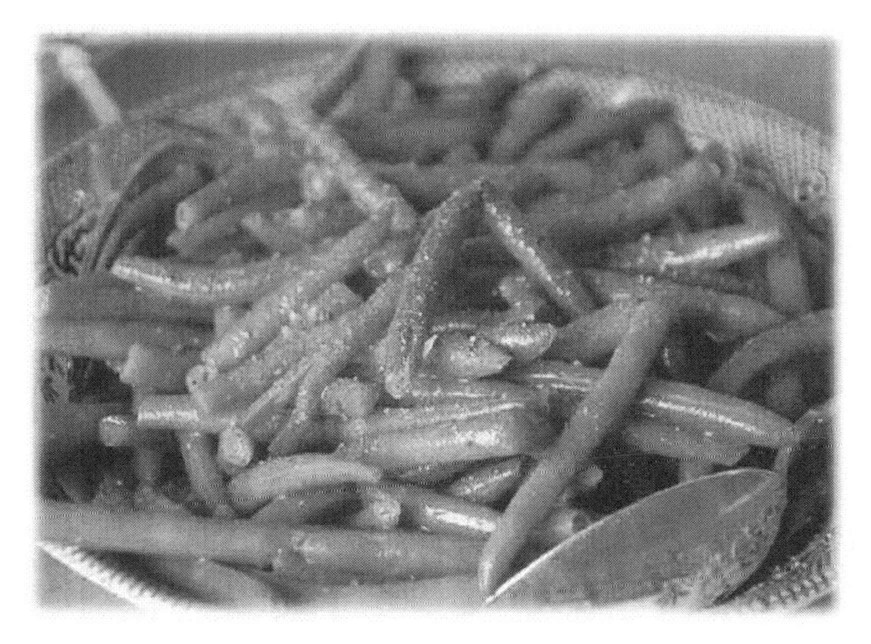

GREEN-BEANS A-LA VERVE

1-pound fresh green beans
MSG-free vegetable stock
Seasonings

Cut string beans tips.
Barely-cover beans in pot of water.
Add vegetable stock and seasonings (salt, pepper, garlic powder).
Boil for 20 minutes.
Separate the stock and drink this nutritious broth.
Eat more to your heart's delight.

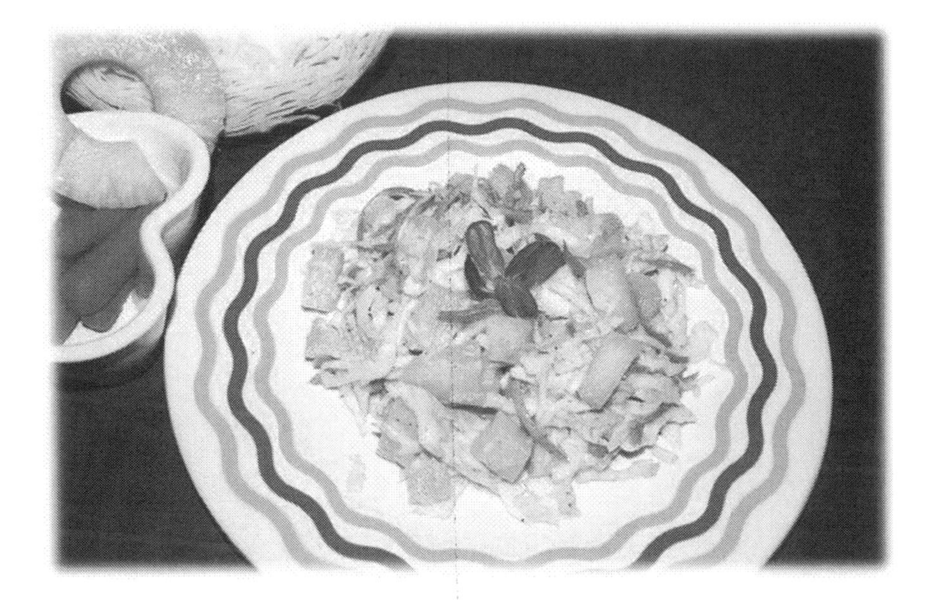

PINEAPPLE SLAW

½ cup olive oil
½ cup pine nuts
3 tablespoons raw honey
1 tablespoon stevia
4 tablespoons apple cider vinegar
½ tablespoon basil
1 large bag (8 cups) slaw mix
1 cup fresh pineapple slices

Mix above ingredients (except slaw and pineapple) in blender.
Pour into large bowl; add slaw and mix well by hand.
Add sea salt to taste then blend in pineapple slices.
Chill for at least one hour.

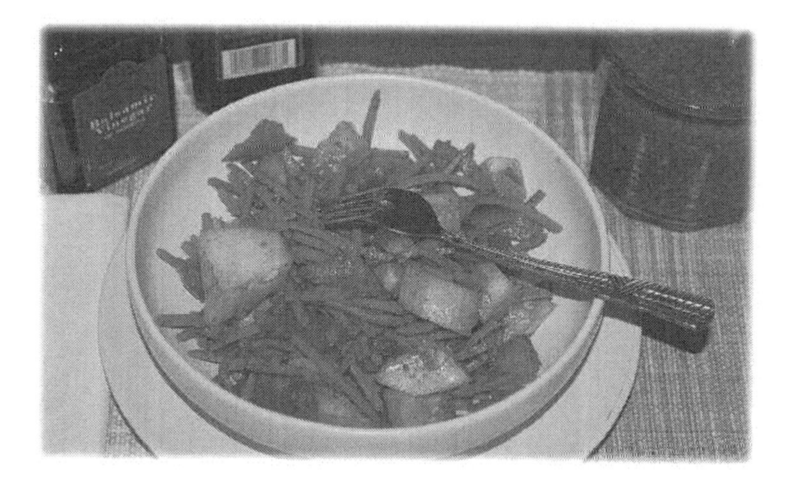

TOMATO-CUKE SALAD

Cut tomatoes, cucumbers and carrots as desired.
Mix balsamic vinegar, olive and seasons to taste.
Garnish with parmesan cheese and/or
Diced raw sweet onion.

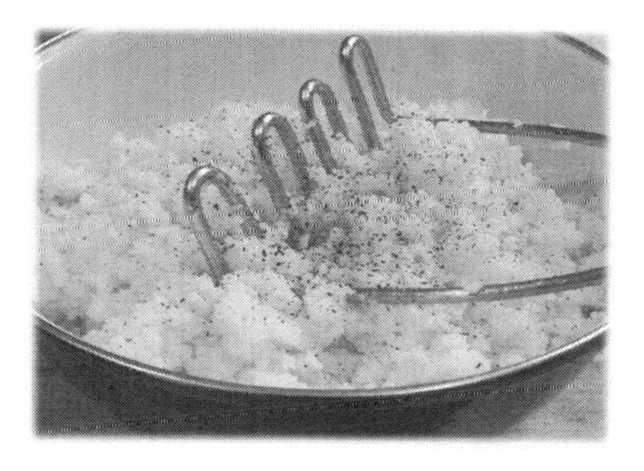

CAULIFLOWER RICE-POTATOES

Boil cauliflower until slightly softened (3-5 minutes).
Mash and season with butter, salt and pepper.
Substitute white potatoes or rice with this delicious
vitamin C-rich vegetable.

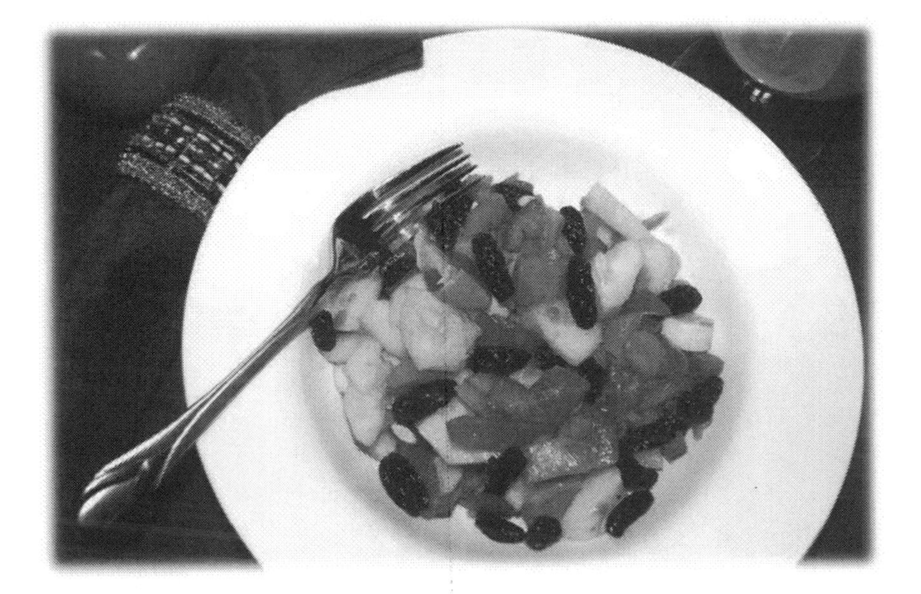

<u>**SWEET-SOUR RAISIN SALAD**</u>

4 hearts-of-palm
1 cucumber
2 tomatoes
10 baby carrots
Raisins

Chop above ingredients by hand or processor.
Marinate in sweet-sour dressing for at least one hour.
Garnish with raisins.

<u>**Sweet-Sour dressing**</u>

½ cup olive oil
2 tablespoons apple cider vinegar
2 tablespoons raw honey

Blend above ingredients.

The key to health by eating as much of the above foods that you want is found not only in eating vitamin packed carbohydrates, but includes eliminating processed and nutrient-depleted foods. This means avoiding starchy and less nutritious vegetables such as peas, corn, beans (except green beans), white potatoes and all canned food with the exception of stewed tomatoes, sugar-free apple sauce and hearts of palm.

Frozen carbohydrates are out; freezing destroys the B and C vitamins. Finally, until your health, vitality and optimum body weight is restored, avoid all grains – not one bite! This means *all* rice and flour-based products (bread, cake, cookies, pancakes, bagels, pasta, etc.).

If you are craving flour and want to cheat, then try to hand mill whole wheat or barley grains at home. An alternative is almond flour. Even so, hand milled grains and almond flour-based goodies will oppose more than help the process of health restoration – so try to wait until you're feeling better before eating grains again.

ELIMINATE:

Starchy Vegetables	**No peas, corn, beans or white potatoes**
Canned and Frozen Vegetables	**Few exceptions**
Grains	**Not one bite!**

"I saw few die of hunger; of eating, a hundred thousand."
-B. Franklin

Step 3: Eat Tryptophan-rich Protein

Tryptophan, an essential amino acid that cells cannot make, is found in dietary protein and is an important nutrient for optimizing health. Serotonin (for good mood), melatonin (for uninterrupted sleep) and dopamine (for clear focus) are brain-based neurotransmitters made from tryptophan, vitamin B6 and magnesium. With sufficient nutrients, cells can also convert tryptophan into nicotinic acid (to make NAD for energy). Mood swings, difficulty thinking, frequent awakenings at the night and/or low energy levels all signal a tryptophan deficiency.

Step Three: Eat tryptophan-rich protein.

Fish, Poultry, Eggs	**Dish it up!**
Batter-dipped frying	***Don't do it!***
AVOID:	**Red meat, pork and bottom-feeders**

Excellent protein sources of tryptophan (from highest to lowest) include eggs, fish, turkey and chicken. These protein-based foods are not only rich in tryptophan, but they are easy to digest and full of vitamins and minerals (the same cannot be said of pork, red meats, farm raised fish and bottom-feeders such as oysters, clams, shrimp and lobster).

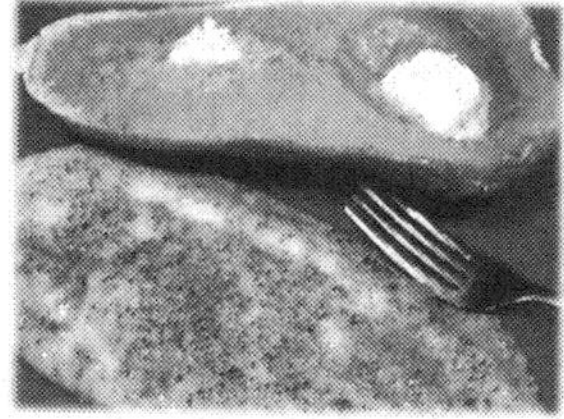

Fish and chicken can be lightly coated with seasonings and baked, grilled or pan-fried with coconut, safflower and/or sesame oil (I use a 50/50 mix of safflower and sesame oil). One or two side dishes of C-foods from Step Two will complete an "all you can eat" healthy meal. Tuna fish salad or chicken salad stuffed inside cleaned cucumbers cut lengthwise, make delicious and tryptophan-rich power meals and a great brown bag it lunch.

Despite all the misinformation and bad press, eggs are one of the most wholesome and healthful sources of protein. Yolk is rich in lecithin which is an important nutrient for normal brain, nerve and cell membrane function. And while egg yolk contains cholesterol, it is not cholesterol in food that makes high blood cholesterol, because all foods are broken down in the stomach and small intestine into molecules much smaller than cholesterol. The liver converts these molecules into cholesterol and releases it into the blood for the rest of the cells in the body to use. High cholesterol in the blood signals that cholesterol is being damaged by oxidation and the liver is busy replacing it (see: "How Statin Drugs Really Lower Cholesterol *And Kill You One Cell at a Time*"). Cholesterol does not come from the food you eat; rather, the food you eat is *made into* cholesterol!

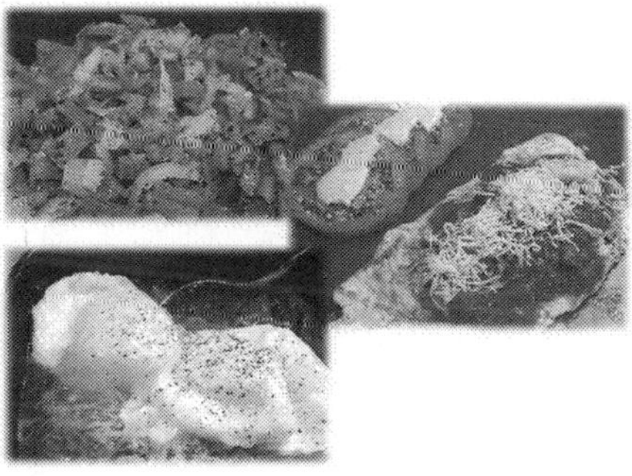

Prepare eggs any way you like, but try to always include raw onions and tomatoes. Omelette fillers include sautéed and raw onions, peppers, tomatoes and most any other vegetable with sliced turkey or turkey sausage for meat lovers. Salsa is an excellent topping on eggs, and a light garnishing with cheese provides an additional source of tryptophan. A side of sliced raw tomatoes will fill the empty spot of what used to be toast, grits or home-fries. Poached eggs atop a bowl of chili with cheese is another creative way to load up on tomatoes in the morning. And don't forget that side of fresh squeezed apple-citrus juice (Step One) to start the day!

"Health alone is victory."
-Thomas Carlyle

Step 4: Get the Skinny on Fat

Half of the fats in cell membranes are saturated with hydrogen (solid oils) and the other half is unsaturated (liquid oils). Two-thirds of unsaturated oils are omega-6 type fats and one-third is omega-3 type fats. Your diet, then, should reflect the same ratio.

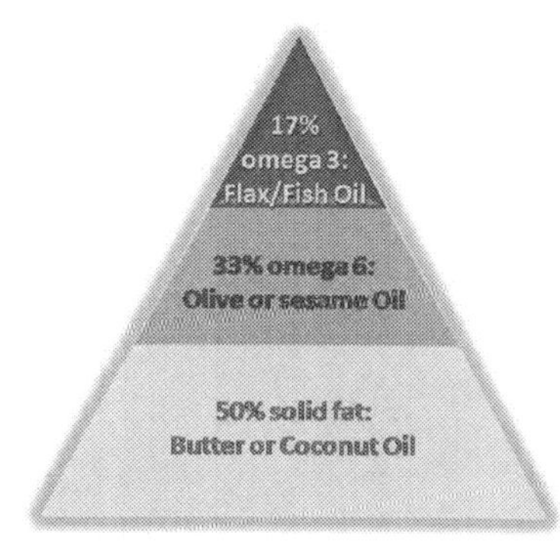

Eating energizing fats in proper balance will be as easy as 1-2-3 if every day you use 1 part flax (or fish) oil, 2 parts olive oil and 3 parts coconut oil and/or butter as follows:

1 Tablespoon of flax oil mixed in cottage cheese or yogurt
2 Tablespoons of olive oil for salads or to sauté
3 Tablespoons of coconut oil to fry and butter to flavor or bake

Step Four: Get the skinny on fat.

Cold Pressed	Coconut, olive and sesame oils
Hydrogenated Anything	*Not for your life!*
AVOID:	Vegetable oil, canola oil, margarine and shortening

If you can stomach a spoonful of cod liver oil, then let the medicine go down! If not, you can try fish oil supplements or eat more omega-3-rich fish such as salmon. Whether you choose fish oil or flax oil as a dietary supplement, omega-3 oils are more-easily absorbed through the small intestine if they are mixed with an emulsifying protein such as cottage cheese or yoghurt. Our favorite omega-3 oil is Barlean's flax oil; this light and essential oil provides a medium for electrons to freely move and thus literally delivers life to cell membranes. Here's our formula:

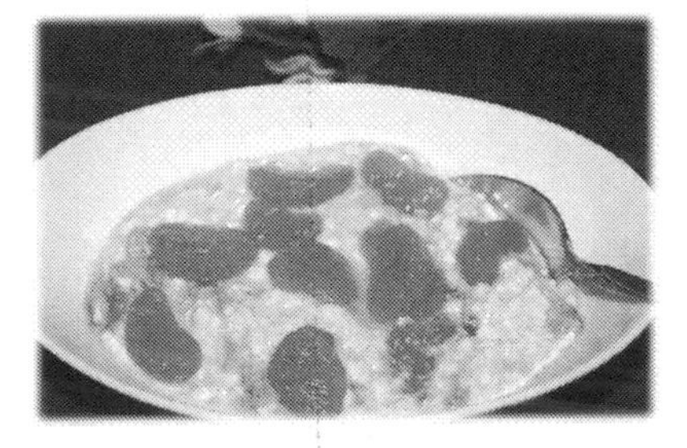

FLAX FIESTA

2 tablespoons Barlean's high lignan flax oil
½ cup cottage cheese
Optional: Mandarin oranges

Mix flax oil with cottage cheese until well-mixed.
Optional: Top with fruit such as mandarin oranges, unsweetened apple sauce or stir-fried diced apples cooked in water and seasoned with cinnamon and stevia.

"The greatest of follies is to sacrifice health for other pleasures.
-Arthur Schopenhauer

Step 5: Snack on Brain Food

While an apple a day keeps the doctor away, six or more apples per day is the best health insurance to keep you away from doctors for life. There is no better energy boosting and health ensuring food than apples.

Apples are metabolic rocket fuel. Malic acid in apples directly boosts the citric acid cycle and propels metabolism forward. This is because malic acid oxidizes to oxaloacetic acid – which is not found in food – which in turn combines with acetyl-CoA to make citric acid to blast the citric acid cycle like rocket fuel! ***Since one of the sources of acetyl-CoA is body fat, malic acid paves the way for more acetyl-CoA from fat to melt away into hydrogen and ATP.*** And the more ATP your brain has to perform its many demanding functions, the fewer food cravings it will generate.

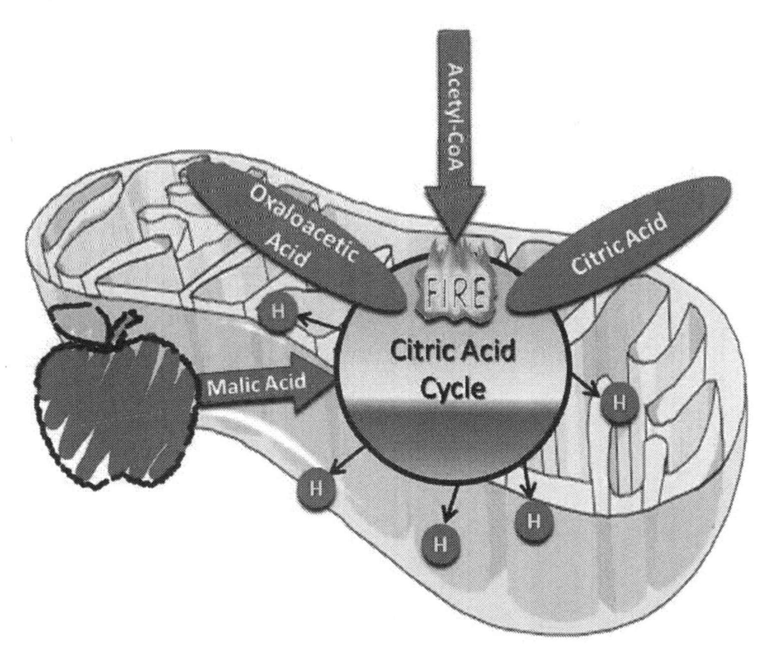

All apples are not the same as some peels are bitter and some fruit sweeter than others. I like Pink Lady, Gala and Fuji. Raw is always preferable to get the most nutrients per sweet bite. Sliced apples doused with fresh squeezed orange juice prevents browning (oxidation). A few cheese slices with fresh apple slices are always a popular taste combination. Cottage cheese mixed with stir-fried apple slices (cooked in a bit of water with cinnamon and raw sugar to taste to make chunky apple sauce) is also a favorite apple/cheese snack combination (add a squeeze of flax oil; your nerves will thank you). Goat cheese and goat's milk, are also excellent protein sources of tryptophan – the wonder molecule that makes you feel good, sleep well and think clearly.

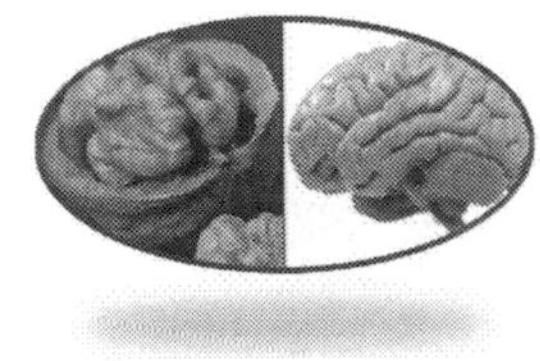

Raw nuts and seeds are a tasty addition to apple and cheese slices. Nuts and seeds are rich in minerals and B-vitamins which also fuel the cellular energy cycle. One of the most important nutrients in nuts and seeds (such as raw pumpkin seeds and sunflower seeds) is *phosphorus* which cells need to make ATP from ADP. While some health nuts insist that roasting nuts does not lower the nutritional content, I've found that roasted nuts do raise blood glucose levels in diabetics *but raw nuts do not*.

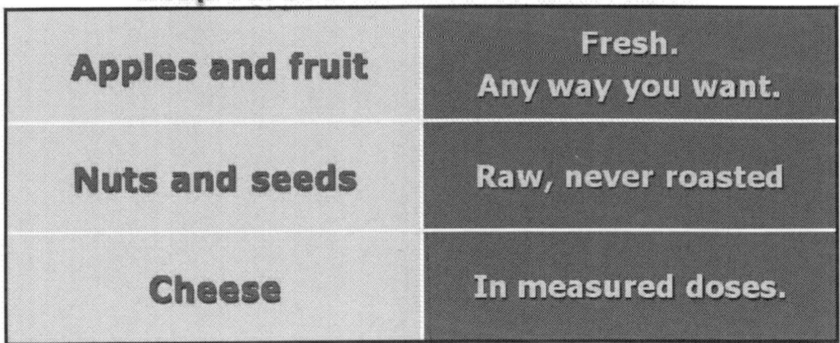

Step Five: Snack on brain food.

Apples and fruit	Fresh. Any way you want.
Nuts and seeds	Raw, never roasted
Cheese	In measured doses.

Some nuts actually look like the brain – small wonder they're such excellent brain food! In place of chips and crackers, keep a ready supply of *raw* walnuts, pecans, cashews and almonds mixed with iodized sea salt to satisfy hunger cravings and provide a quick source of energy. Raisins, dried apple and dates are a naturally sweet addition.

If you find you're craving old favorites such as crackers or bread, “Wasa” bread makes a healthful treat (up to 6 slices per day). For a garnish, try chopped cabbage, sweet onions, peppers and spices boiled in broth until soft. And for those tangerines on the snack plate…eat more not less!

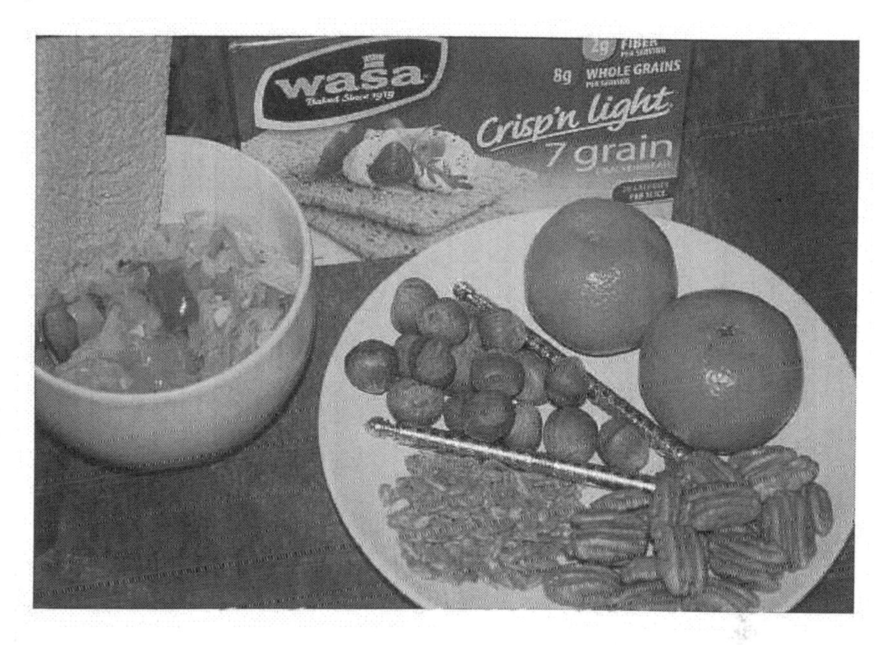

“A man too busy to care for his health is like a mechanic who ruins his tools.”

-Spanish Proverb

Step 6: Maintain Your Batteries

Since ATP is the ultimate fuel that energizes every cell in your body, it only makes sense to continually support the ATP producing factories: the mighty mitochondria.

There are three ways to support those peanut-shaped batteries:

1. Drink chlorine/fluoride-free mineral rich water and freshly made fruit juice (preferably unrefrigerated).

2. Eat nutrient-rich carbs hat thoroughly oxidize into hydrogen to make ATP.

3. Choose fats and supplements that make healthy membranes and therefore healthy mitochondria.

The foods and fats recommended (and banned) in steps one through five are all designed to support your batteries. Two additional food supplements will further ensure optimum mitochondrial health: Collagen boosters and vitamin-mineral supplements.

Step Six: Maintain your batteries.

Collagen boosters	Ascorbic acid, lysine and proline
Multi-vitamin Multi-mineral	A,B,C,D,E Calcium and magnesium
Nicotinic acid	NADH, NAD or Nutritional Yeast

Collagen is the glue that knits cells, tissues and organs together. It strengthens everything! ***Weak nails, thinning skin, bleeding gums, spider veins on the face, poor blood flow and sore joints are just a few of a many symptoms due to "falling apart at the seams" from a collagen deficiency.*** So help pull yourself and your mitochondria together by taking a daily supplement mix of powdered ascorbic acid (Vitamin C), powdered lysine and powdered proline as these three nutrients work together to make collagen (proline and lysine are building blocks of protein). All of these supplements are available at most health food and vitamin stores. Simply mix the ingredients as directed in fresh-squeezed juice every day.

The protein complex imbedded in the inner mitochondrial membrane is dense with certain minerals such as iron, copper and zinc which allow electrons to freely move. Raw nuts and seeds are some of the best natural sources of these minerals.

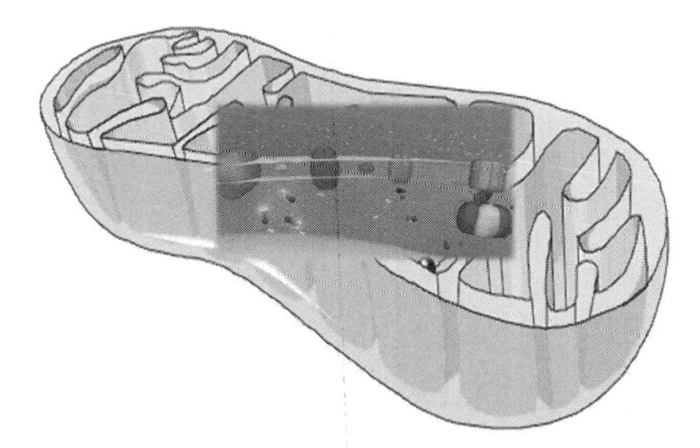

Because current farming methods deplete soils of minerals normally absorbed by plants, I recommend a daily multi-vitamin/mineral supplement, preferably in a gel cap form (rather than tablet or capsule form) as gel caps are more easily reabsorbed through the intestines. Liquid vitamin and mineral supplements, while well absorbed, are usually made with sugar or unhealthy sugar substitutes like Splenda.

Mitochondria are bathed in cell water, and operate most efficiently in a basic pH. Daily calcium and magnesium supplements help ensure your body water maintains a healthy basic pH. Additionally, these minerals are involved in many of the biochemical reactions that occur within mitochondria. Calcium citrate (with vitamin D for enhanced absorption) and magnesium malate are excellent daily sources of these minerals, in tablet or capsule form. This is because the *citrate* (or citric acid) in calcium citrate and *malate* (or malic acid) in magnesium malate both directly fuel the citric acid cycle. Other less effective forms of magnesium (such as magnesium oxide) can cause diarrhea, which is generally not the case with magnesium malate. Furthermore, other forms of calcium (such as calcium carbonate) are not as readily absorbed into cells as calcium citrate.

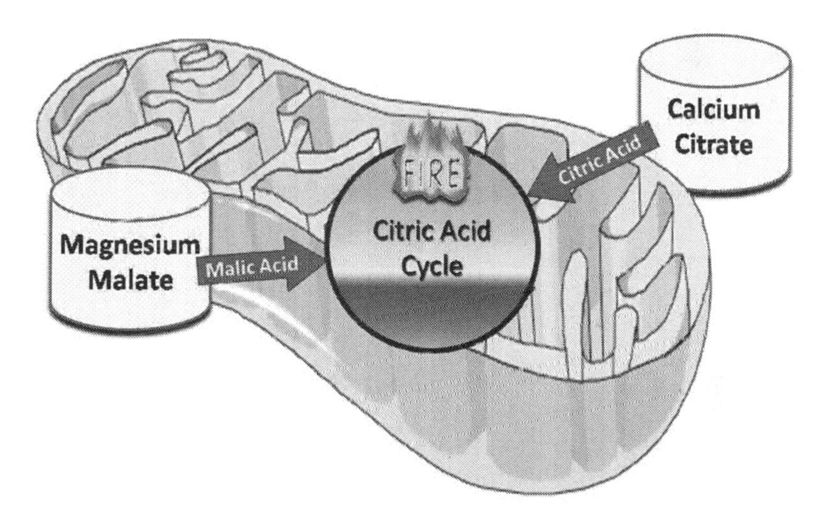

Last, and by all means not least, is daily supplementation of nicotinic acid, which is so readily destroyed by modern food processing methods. Nicotinic acid is used by liver cells to make NAD, which is directly involved in making 80% of the potential energy made by mitochondria. Wow! That's an important nutrient, then, to make sure you have a plentiful supply of every day. Because it is water-soluble and passes through the urine, you need a regular source of NAD.

Nicotinic acid can be supplemented with NAD or NADH tablets (or lozenges) which are all available at health food and vitamin stores. ***If apples are the "rocket fuel" of carbs, then NAD and NADH are the "rocket fuel" of food supplements.*** People plagued with chronic fatiguing conditions such as ALS have reported significant improvement in energy and clarity of thought with two simple supplements: NAD and magnesium malate (malate comes from apples).

Some people report a noticeable increase in energy (without any negative side effects) within 30 minutes of taking an NADH supplement, followed by fatigue early in the afternoon. This can be corrected by taking half of a tablet in the morning with breakfast, and taking the other half in the afternoon with lunch. NAD is a slightly different formulation than NADH, and some people have reported better results with NAD. NAD and NADH should not cause facial flushing, itching or liver problems.

To sum: A collagen-making powdered mix, one multi-vitamin/multi-mineral gel cap, magnesium malate, calcium citrate and a daily source of nicotinic acid (NAD or NADH) will ensure mitochondria have the necessary nutrients to perform their demanding ATP-making function.

All supplements should be taken with food because they are, after all, *food* supplements and perform their function in helping to oxidize the food you eat which, in turn, makes energy for life.

"Our health always seems more precious when it's gone."
-Anonymous

Step 7: Don't be Fooled by Fake Foods

Most people dread the four-letter-word "diet" because of what they must give up rather than what they get to eat. In an effort to replace favorite fat and acid forming foods, many buy into food and drink replacements that they believe will help them only to find they lose more health.

One of the biggest fat lies in the food industry is the "fat-free" label on many tasty and fat-promoting processed grains. All carbohydrates are converted into the sugar glucose by the liver. The label "fat-free" is a misleading half truth. As you now know, it is not fat in food that makes one fat; rather, it is processed nutrient-poor carbohydrates – which are sugars – that make fat. Cookies, cakes, candies and chips that are made without oil, butter or shortening are all "fat free" – and will make just as much waste fat and acids as the same recipes made with fat!

Step Seven: Don't be fooled by fake foods.

"Fat-free"	Big fat lie.
"Low calorie"	Counting calories is bunk.
"Sugar-free" or "Diet"	A sure-fire way to get super-sized and sick.

Processed white sugar, for example, is indeed "fat-free" – but it is also "nutrient-free." Since white sugar doesn't have one iota of vitamins or minerals in it, once ingested it is like wet wood on a fire. It might burn to acetyl-CoA only to face eviction from the mitochondria and converted to fat in the cell water, because it doesn't carry with it the nutrients that are needed to burn into hydrogen in the citric acid cycle. If you added some white sugar, on the other hand, to fresh squeezed apple-citrus juice that's loaded with vitamins and minerals, the nutrient-rich juice would likely contain enough vitamins to oxidize the sugar. The trade-off is that the juice will have less energy-making power than if it had been made without the sugar. The nutrients are wasted to burn the sugar rather than to burn stored fat. Don't do it.

Low calorie processed foods that have been stripped of vitamins are another big fat lie. ***Counting calories is bunk.*** Reading the vitamins on food labels is also a waste of time, because manufactured vitamins can be added to foods to make them *look* nutritious. Adding man-made vitamins to processed grains, or any man-manipulated food, is never a substitute for natural vitamins found in fresh foods. Furthermore, vitamin B3 is almost always supplemented in the wrong form as niacinamide rather than nicotinic acid – and it is the latter which cells preferentially use to make NAD to make ATP.

Finally, diet soda is one of the most disease promoting drinks in the world. Nothing you drink will make you more fatigued and sick than diet soda. The pH-lowering effect of soda not only robs your cells of alkaline minerals such as calcium, it lowers the pH of everything, compromises oxidation and feeds acid-loving cholesterol-robbing CWD bacteria.

Drinking diet soda is a sure-fire way to get sick, sore and even super-sized.

"The first wealth is health."
-Ralph Waldo Emerson

Step 8: If You Can't Read it, Don't Eat it

Approval of a food or food additive by the FDA is no guarantee of its safety. FDA approval is usually based upon what is revealed to them by manufacturers and information gleaned from short term studies. Serious safety issues do not usually come to light until a product has been in the market for some time, and even then, cause and effect connections between illness and a food product might never be made. Soda is one example.

Step Eight: If you can't read it, *don't eat it.*

Sugar substitutes	Danger!
"PPG/PEG"	This is antifreeze!
Some colors and preservatives	Poison!

Keep it simple. If you can't pronounce a word on the ingredients label of any processed food, *don't buy it*! And if by chance you can pronounce it but you don't know what it is, *look it up*! Take control of your health and never blindly ignore labels by blindly trusting that the FDA has thoroughly done their homework. FDA employees are just as susceptible to being conned by hidden agendas of big business as the rest of us. The FDA, after all, approved statins.

Before medical school, I worked as an applications engineer for an evaporator manufacturer of specialty heat exchangers made out of titanium and stainless steel. When customers chose city water as the source of heat for their equipment, we were adamant that all fluoride and chloride (halogen) molecules had to be completely removed from the water prior to allowing it into the heat exchanger. Otherwise, the stainless steel and titanium would be "etched" (degraded) by these electron robbing chemicals. Halogens are strong oxidizers which degrade some of the strongest metals on earth such as titanium – and yet humans ingest poisons that degrade metal! If chlorine isn't safe for titanium, you can be pretty sure that it's not safe for you. Protect your electron-rich membranes and myelin sheathes!

DO NOT DRINK CHLORINATED WATER – EVER!!

Deodorants contain aluminum and antifreeze (PPG or PEG), both of which are also highly toxic to cells. The axillary lymph nodes notably drain from the underarm to the upper-outer portion of the breast where the majority of breast tumors are found. Find a natural substitute.

Here's a top-ten list of toxic additives to avoid:

"GMO" or "Modified." These are genetically modified organisms, found mostly in corn and soy products. "Modified" corn starch, for example, is a GMO product. GMO foods are outlawed in health-conscious countries like New Zealand. Think like a health savvy Kiwi and say "no" to GMO. These are fit for Frankenstein but not for you.

Sucralose (Splenda) and Saccharine (Equal). These toxic sweeteners are neither splendid nor equal to raw sugar. Safe alternatives to raw sugar include xylitol and stevia.

Fructose Corn Syrup (and High Fructose Corn Syrup). This is a commercially-made, unnatural sugar found in many processed foods. It taxes the liver which must convert fructose to glucose and then robs the body of its nutrient treasures because it contains no vitamins or minerals. Furthermore, these syrups are made from genetically modified corn.

PPG/PEG. This is found in underarm deodorants and foods such as cream cheese, vanilla flavored extracts and salad dressings. PPG is poly-propylene glycol and PPE is poly-ethylene glycol which is highly toxic *antifreeze*. A small amount of PEG, for example, will quickly kill a small animal. An informed veterinarian treating a pet with rapidly failing kidneys will ask the pet owner if he or she has recently changed the radiator water in their car and dumped it on the ground (animals lick it from the ground because it smells and tastes sweet). If a few licks kill a cat, it's not good for you!

MSG and hydrolyzed protein. Hydrolyzed proteins like MSG are used to enhance flavor. These adulterated proteins are as unnatural as hydrogenated oils and are frequently found in sauces (such as soy sauce) and soups. Soy sauce (and saki) is also made by fermenting a cancer causing fungus (liver cancer is the number one cause of death in the East). "Bragg's liquid aminos" (found at health food stores) is made with essential amino acids from non-hydrolyzed protein and is an excellent substitute for soy sauce.

Nitrites. This preservative, found in many processed meats such as hotdogs and sausages, has long been linked with stomach cancer.

Dyes and Colorings. These are found in many processed foods with poor nutritional value and should be avoided as some dyes are carcinogenic. Blue #1, blue #2, red #3, green #3 and yellow #6 cause cancer in lab animals. These dyes are also common in pet food. Your dog does not care about the color of his crunchy nuggets and chew hides.

Olestra. This fake FDA approved fat causes cramps, loose stools and inhibits absorption of the fat-soluble vitamins (A, D, E and K).

Potassium bromate and TBHQ. Potassium bromate adds volume to breads. TBHQ is a popcorn preservative. Both cause cancer in lab animals.

Hard-to-read-words. If you can't pronounce it, don't buy it.

Bottom line:

- ***IF YOU CAN'T READ IT, DON'T EAT IT!***
- ***IF YOU DON'T KNOW WHAT IT IS, TOSS IT!***
- ***IF IT CAN SIT ON A SHELF IN A BOX OR BAG FOR MORE THAN A MONTH, THINK TWICE!***

What kind of cornball idea is it to ingest any poison in any amount regardless of claims to safety? If the FDA ever approves a dash of CN to go with FDA-approved titanium dioxide (floor finish) as cake preservative, you might want to know what it was that took away all your breath.

"What is called genius is the abundance of life and health."
-Henry David Thoreau

Step 9: Avoid Center Aisles for Your Life

The center aisles of a grocery store, in general, are where you can find the stock of processed foods that are not *real* foods. They are empty calories that can sit on shelves for years because they contain no active B or C vitamins that oxidize and spoil food. Many of these scrumptious fares are made from stripped grains such as wheat and rice. This includes pasta, breads, crackers, cereals, chips, bagels, cookies, muffins, cakes, pies and "instant" mixes of rice and various noodle concoctions.

Calculating the calories of these non-foods makes as much sense as weighing wet wood for a fire. Wet wood is wet wood, and whether light or heavy it simply doesn't burn well. Similarly, the calories of processed grains mean nothing in regards to energy value. Calories mean nothing because key vitamins and minerals are the measure of what oxidizes food into energy. Fifty calories of fat-making chips simply makes fifty calories of fat and 500 calories of fat-making chips makes 500 calories of fat.

Most cereals made with oats and barley have been polished, steamed, crushed, rolled, puffed and popped; say "so-long" to the heat-sensitive B vitamins that are so essential to carbohydrate oxidation. Even grape-nuts and brans seem to promote weight gain.

Frozen foods are essentially dead weight like wet wood. This includes ice creams, frozen yoghurt and sherbets which are loaded with fructose corn syrup, sugar substitutes, gums and preservatives. The only food worth reaching for in a grocer's freezer is fish, but even fresh fish is preferable to frozen.

Canned and jarred foods are rarely additive-free and have few vitamins due to heat pasteurization. Exceptions include apple sauce without sugar, stewed whole and crushed tomatoes (*not* tomato sauce which usually contains fructose corn syrup), coconut milk, almond milk, beans, chick peas, hearts of palm and most anything with only one ingredient that is a natural food.

Step Nine: Avoid center aisles for your life.

Boxed foods	Rarely
Frozen foods	Exception: Fish
Cans and jars	Few exceptions

With few exceptions, grocery store center aisles are dead food zones. Avoid these. They are imitations of food that will titillate your taste buds but tamper with your health.

"Let nothing treatable by diet be treated by other means."
-Maimonides

Step 10: Don't Desert Dessert

Once you're feeling stronger and more energized, you may want to spice up life a bit with some healthy desserts. Fruit is always the best choice for a naturally sweet AND nutritious dessert.

Strange, but sadly true, many doctors recommend that diabetics not eat fruit because it is high in sugar! It is *not* sugar in fruit that makes blood sugar high; rather, it is vitamin-deficient carbohydrates that elevate blood sugar – and fresh fruits are packed with active vitamins! In ***fact, raw honey, apples and citrus*** are some of the most potent foods (medicines) for normalizing elevated blood sugar. Honey is so effective at lowering blood glucose, that if you tend to have low blood sugar (hypoglycemia), you may want to avoid it.

Sorbet is a tasty substitute for store bought ice cream, frozen yoghurt and sherbet which are all tainted with corn syrup, sugar-substitutes, preservatives and gummy additives. A delicious but hard-to-find fruit called "sapote" (pronounced *sah-po-tay*) can be substituted in these recipes with strawberries. All of these delicious deserts can be enjoyed without adding waste acids to your water. Some take a bit of time to prepare, but the payoff is health and long life. Enjoy!

Step Ten: Don't desert dessert.

Fresh fruit	Naturally-sweet
Ice cream/sherbet	Make fresh sorbet!
Baked goods	Try dehydrating instead.

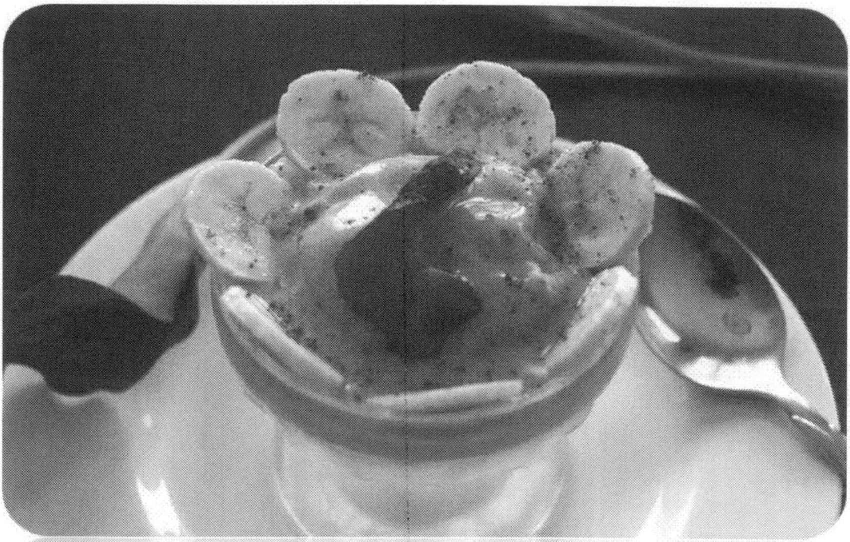

Strawberry Sorbet

32 oz. almond milk
14 oz can coconut milk
40 frozen strawberries
2 bananas
4 tablespoons honey
8 packets stevia

Mix above ingredients in blender.
Freeze for 1-2 hours until soft-frozen.
Garnish with banana and strawberry.
Sprinkle with nutmeg.

Serves 8

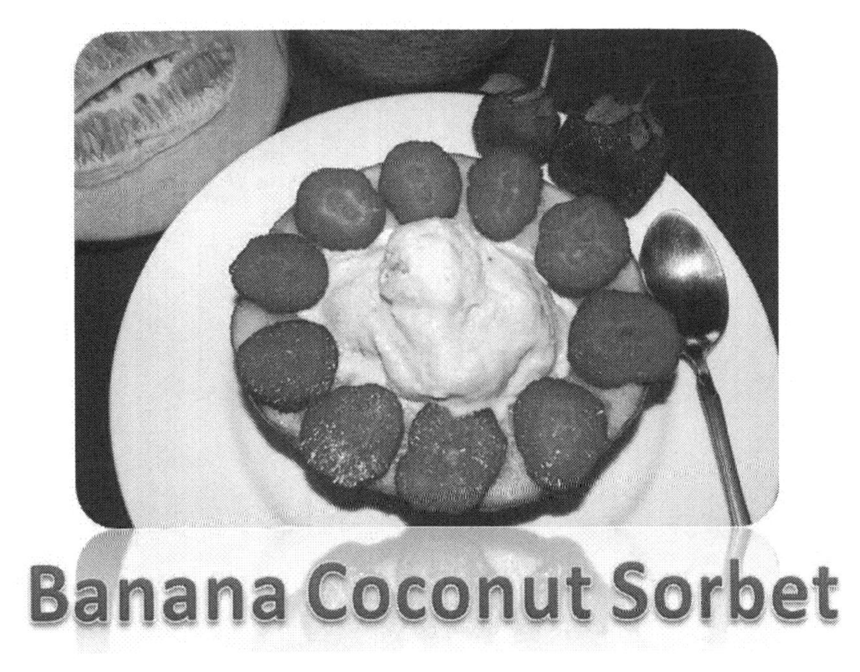

Banana Coconut Sorbet

14 oz. can of coconut milk
1 banana
¼ teaspoon cinnamon
2 teaspoons vanilla extract
6 soaked dates with outer skin removed
6 packets stevia

Mix above ingredients in blender.
Freeze for 3-4 hours until soft-frozen.
Serve in de-seeded cantaloupe.
Garnish strawberries with stevia.

Serves 2

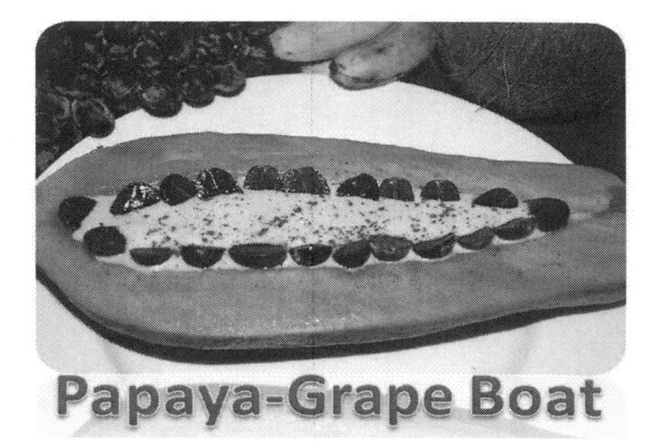

Use the same recipe as above for Banana Coconut Sorbet but:
Substitute 6 strawberries for 6 dates and serve in papaya.
Garnish with grapes.

Serves 2

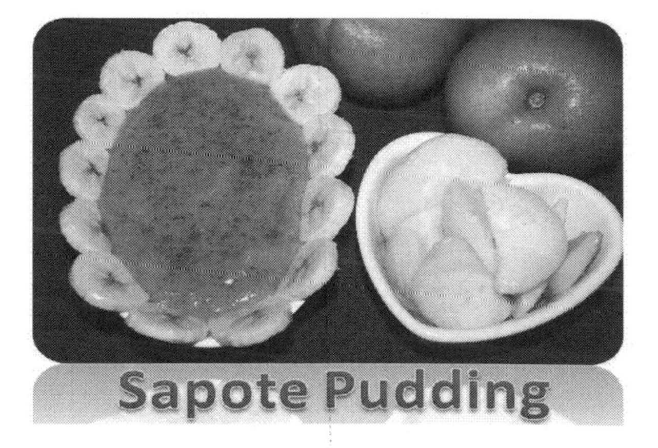

1 sapote and 1 banana
(May substitute sapote with 3 strawberries)
1 teaspoon pure vanilla extract

Mix above ingredients in blender and serve.
Garnish with cinnamon and banana.

Serves 2

Dehydration is a low temperature (below 140°F) cooking method that preserves heat-sensitive vitamins. Dehydrated apple and banana slices chew like candy, and liquefied bananas poured onto non-stick sheets will dehydrate to make delicious fruit roll-ups. The *Excalibur* tray-style dehydrator is an excellent unit, large enough to accommodate batches of fruits, vegetables and even meats for making jerky. You can "process" your own vegetables by dehydration and storing them in vacuum-sealed plastic bags to have at-the-ready to rehydrate in soups and stews; these will last for years. The denser the vegetable (less water), the better the result. This includes sliced: sweet potatoes, onions, garlic, mushrooms and carrots. Men love the jerky, kids enjoy the roll-ups and, because the possibilities are endless, food dehydration projects pulls the whole family together in the creative process of preparing whole foods.

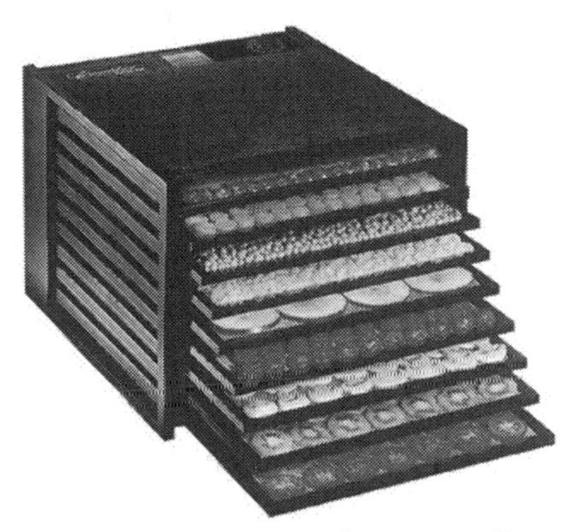

Here's a few delicious and nutritious dehydration creations that draw plenty of comments like, "We've never seen *this* before!"

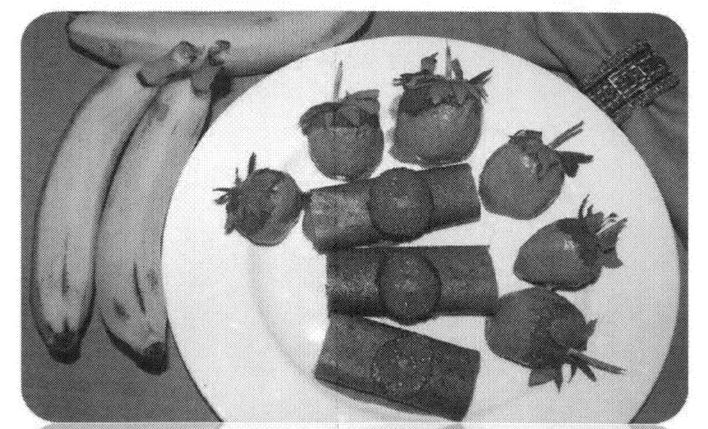

Banana Date Nut Crepes

Banana Crepe Roll

Mix four bananas in blender and spread thin onto non-stick dehydrator tray liners.
Dehydrate for 10-12 hours at 120ºF.
Turn after 6-8 hours and remove tray liners.
Cut into 3-inch wide, 5-inch long pieces.

Banana-Date-Nut Filling

2 tablespoons almond butter
2 bananas
10 soaked dates with outer skin removed
¼ teaspoon cinnamon and ¼ teaspoon vanilla extract
Dash of nutmeg

Mix above ingredients in blender.
Place in freezer for 15 minutes.
Fill crepes with banana-date-nut filling and roll each crepe.
Dip whole strawberries with leftover dip.
Garnish with sliced strawberries.

Serves 2

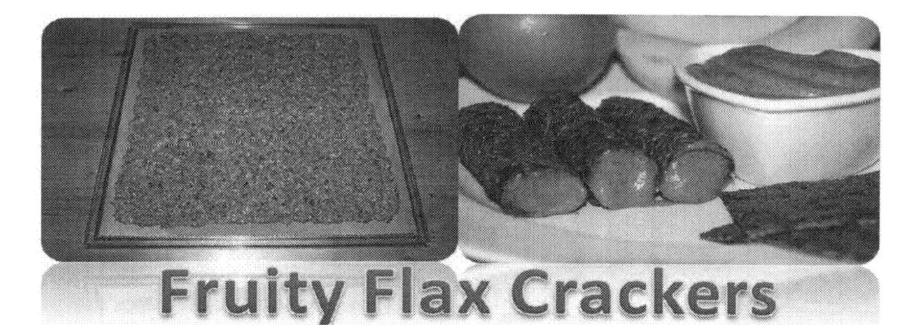

Fruity Flax Crackers

2 cups golden flax seed
(soak flax seed in 2 cups water for 2 hours)
½ cup soaked dates (outer skins removed)
½ cup soaked apricots
½ cup raisins
1 banana

Blend above ingredients in food processor.
Spread onto non-stick dehydrator tray liners (about 1/8 inch thick).
Dehydrate for 10-12 hours at 120°F.
Turn after 6-8 hours and remove tray liners.
Break or cut into 3" x 4" crackers.

Makes two trays.

<u>Banana-Sapote Filling</u>

1 banana and 1 sapote
(or substitute sapote with 3 strawberries)
½ cup soaked chopped dates
2 tablespoons almond butter
1 tablespoon raw honey
½ tablespoon cinnamon

Mix above ingredients in blender.
Fill crackers generously with filling and roll.

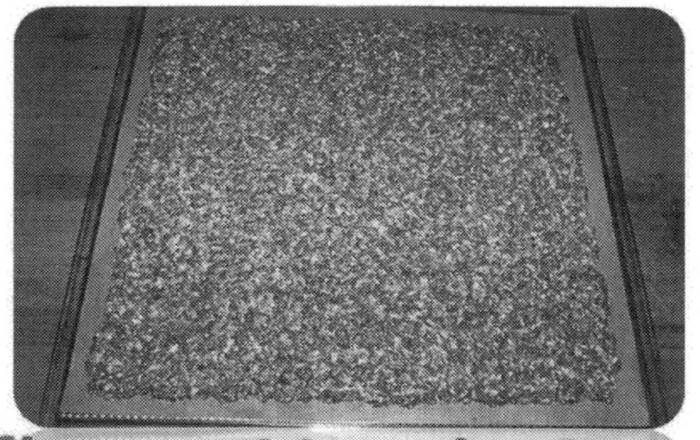

Sunflower Veggie Crackers

3 cups golden flax seed (soak in 3 cups water for 2 hours)
1 cup raw sunflower seeds
6 cups sunflower seed sprouts
1 cup raw pine nuts
2 cloves raw garlic
20 baby carrots
½ red bell pepper
1 tomato
10 soaked sun-dried tomatoes
½ teaspoon hot chili pepper
1 tablespoon oregano
1 tablespoon basil
½ tablespoon Italian seasoning
½ teaspoon sea salt

Grind sunflower seeds in coffee grinder.
Set flax seed and sunflower seed powder aside.
Blend remaining ingredients in processor.
Transfer to large bowl.
By hand, mix in sunflower seed powder and flax seed.
Spread onto non-stick dehydrator tray liners (1/8 inch thick).
Dehydrate for 10-12 hours at 120°F.
Turn after 6-8 hours and remove non-stick liners.

Makes three trays

Epilogue: Pulling it All Together

The ALS diet is the power of hydrogen in water and food:

1. Hydrogen in water: "Less is more". Less hydrogen leaves more oxygen in water to oxidize food efficiently and evict disease causing CWD microbes that hate oxygen.

2. Hydrogen in food (oxidized): "More is better". More hydrogen removed from carbohydrates makes more ATP and leaves fewer waste acids to contaminate your body water.

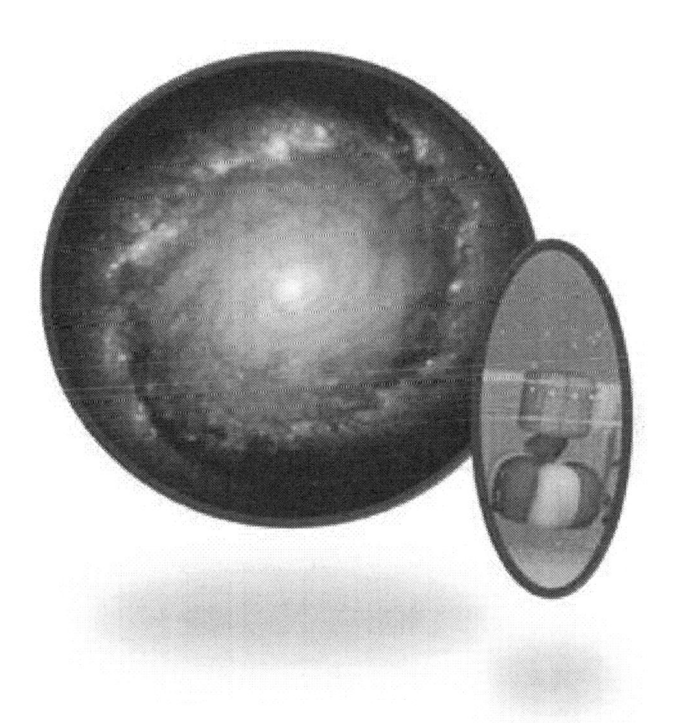

The spin of the ALS diet is all about spinning hydrogen from nutritious carbohydrates that makes lots of ATP and keeps your water clean and well oxygenated.

Beautiful videos of spinning hydrogen making ATP can be found at the Virtual Cell Collection (http://vcell.ndsu.nodak.edu).

Conquering ALS means adopting protocols that are not based upon conjecture but on proven science. That roadmap is this book.

Three virtues are also needed to conquer ALS: patience, hope and rightly-divided trust.

One of the keys to recovery is patience. Chemistry students quickly learn that more is not always better when conducting chemical reactions in a controlled setting. Chronic illnesses don't develop over night and neither does the recovery process.

As you fuel your body with real medicine (real food), there are outward signs that signal cellular health is being restored:

1. Nails will grow faster and become less brittle.
2. A white-coated tongue will become healthy and pink.
3. Dry, dull and thinning hair will become thick and shiny.
4. Thick scaly skin on the knees and elbows will clear up.
5. A butterfly rash will dissipate.
6. Recurrent bladder infections will lessen and stop.
7. Nail fungus will disappear as new nails advance.
8. Bowel function will regulate.
9. Breathlessness will decrease.
10. Muscle strength and endurance will increase.
11. Psychiatric and emotional problems will balance out.
12. Libido will increase.
13. Clarity of thought (focus) and memory will improve.
14. Muscle and joint pain will subside.
15. Grip strength will improve.
16. Teeth sensitivity and bleeding gums will resolve.
17. Hemorrhoids will heal faster, recur less and/or stop.
18. Swollen ankles will improve.
19. Blood pressure will normalize.
20. Ringing in the ears and/or imbalance will decrease.

Is there hope? Yes, but you will not find it in your doctor's office. The practice of medicine has completely lost its way. The search for cures has been replaced by remedies that treat symptoms and only offer some relief. No one noticed.

The problem is much more pervasive and sinister than that. The first and most basic tenant of medicine is "to do no harm". That tenant has been so corrupted by pharmaceutical companies that it no longer plays into the practice of medicine.

Bribes are not necessary. The purchase of influence is done in full public view with consulting fees, honoraria and future jobs in the industry. The drug industry has inserted itself into the NIH, the FDA and virtually every organization that controls medicine. The protocols for treatment are written by physicians at the NIH, AMA, AHA and universities who consult for drug companies. The order of the day is called prevention, not with good nutrition and lifestyle but with drugs of questionable veracity. Statins are only one of those drugs.

The first rule of health must be skepticism, not blind trust. Any food or drug approved by the FDA and recommended by the food or drug industry is questionable. Common sense dictates that if it needed approval, it was questionable in the first place.

To begin a nutritious healing lifestyle requires giving up questionable foods, drugs and drinks. Under the tenet of "do no harm" that is neither difficult nor dangerous.

Chlorinated water must go. It is not coincidental that the advent of runaway chronic degenerative and autoimmune diseases coincides with the chlorination of water. Chlorine turns water into a dangerous oxidizing liquid that eats away at metal pipes over years, even stainless steel and titanium. In the soft lipid-lined arteries that are subject to inhaled and swallowed oxidizers, it is gradually deadly. This fact has been known for at least fifty years.

Tobacco smoke must go. It is another lipid oxidizer.

Soft drinks must also be eliminated. Along with the chlorination of water came Coca Cola and a plethora of fizzy beverages that contain phosphoric acid – another slow death calcium-robbing, oxidizing liquid.

No harm can come from drinking filtered mineral rich spring water.

All dead foods must go. Carbohydrates either turn into acid and fat (anergy) or ATP and health (energy). If a food has been robbed of its nutritional value to prolong its shelf life or make it pretty, do not eat it.

Why do we trust drug companies and the doctors who sell their sometimes snake oil wares? It is clear that we trust – and we do it a lot. We trust our healers. We trust our governments. We trust our pastors and priests. We trust our friends and family, husbands and wives. We trust our pharmacists. We trust ourselves.

Why is trust and being trusted so important to us? We find it insulting to not be trusted; conversely, we fear insulting someone for expressing distrust.

Trust is an irrational emotion. It is the opposite of rational accountability. Accountability is good; trust, alone, is not. With trust comes deceit, corruption and harm. Distrust is as irrational as trust. With distrust come fear, jealousy, paranoia and isolation. Accountability resolves both. With accountability comes trustworthiness.

Trust with accountability is necessary; they mix well when we take complete responsibility for our own trusting. If trust we must, particularly when our lives depend on it, then we must require an accounting of those we trust and hold that they be and remain trustworthy.

Liars, cheats and thieves make victims; conversely, victims make liars, cheats and thieves.

We have a personal responsibility to be skeptical. We also have a personal responsibility to be completely and fully accountable. Accountability is good. Until we are, we cannot hold anyone else's feet to the fire. Oddly the two coincide. We must be held accountable for not being skeptical. Accountability and skepticism make trust work. Nothing else does.

Blind trust never works.

We must stop blindly trusting doctors. Doctors have been trained to chase numbers more than health. Drug companies take advantage of this with chemical trickery to move molecules out of the blood and improve blood lab numbers. The consequences can be deadly. MER/29, Thalidomide, Avandia, Baycol and Vioxx serve as a few examples.

What then can we do? Be wise. Don't quickly buy onto scientific claims made by any companies with a financial interest even if the claims concern an FDA-approved drug or device. Sound science and money never mix. "FDA approval" means something was wrong in the first place.

Always investigate long and confusing constructs. That is a tip-off that something is amiss. Truth of any matter is never beyond one's reach of understanding. Don't be baffled by BS.

Finally, if you have drug-induced ALS from taking a statin drug, know that the difficulty with recovering from statin use is that some damage is slow to heal and other damage may not repair at all and be permanent. No one knows for sure. Consider bringing a copy of "How Statin Drugs Really Lower Cholesterol *And Kill You One Cell at a Time*" to your doctor for a second opinion. He or she, after all, might also be a victim of trust in the medical system and have a second thought about prescribing you or anyone else another statin. If you are a statin-injured victim, consider bringing the same book to your injury lawyer for advisement; he or she may have a second thought about the strength of your "failure to warn" complaint.

If you have the courage and the motivation to get well informed, there is hope. Take charge of your own wellness. Good health is more than physical; it is mental, emotional and spiritual. It is very difficult to be patient, hopeful and a guardian of trust when feeling sick and tired of being sick and tired, especially when one's needs are so demanding. Try it anyway.

The true miracle of humanity is change. We have the capacity to be different than we used to be or were born to be.

Please feel free to share with me your journey on the road to conquering ALS. Take this road map with you and be well.

Much care,

Hannah Yoseph, MD

References

1. Chen W. High Prevalence of Mycoplasma Pneumoniae in Intestinal Mucosal Biopsies from Patients with Inflammatory Bowel Disease and Controls. *Digestive Diseases and Sciences,* 2001: 46 (11): 2529-2535.

2. Roediger W, Macfarlane G. A Role For Intestinal Mycoplasmas in the Etiology of Crohn's dDsease? *Journal of Applied Microbiology,* 2002: 92 (3): 377-381.

3. Matsuo M, Tsuchiya K, Hamasaki Y, Singer H. Restless Legs Syndrome: Association With Streptococcal or Mycoplasma Infection. *Pediatric Neurology,* 2004: 31 (2): 119-21.

4. Reunanen A, Roivainen M, Kleemola M, Saikku P, Leinonen M, Hovi T, Knekt P, Leino A, Aromaa A. Enterovirus, Mycoplasma and Other Infections as Predictors for Myocardial Infarction. *Journal of Internal Medicine,* 2002: 252 (5): 421-429.

5. Rothstein T, Kenny G. Cranial Neuropathy, Myeloradiculopathy, and Myositis: Complications of Mycoplasma. *Internal Medicine,* 1979: 36: 476-477.

6. Haier J, Nasralla M, Franco A, Nicolson G. Detection of Mycoplasmal Infections in Blood of Patients With Rheumatoid Arthritis. *Rheumatology,* 1999: 38: 504–509.

7. Davis C, Cochran S, Lisse J, Buck G, DiNuzzo A, Weber T, Reinarz J. Isolation of Mycoplasma Pneumoniae from Synovial Fluid Samples in a Patient With Pneumonia and Polyarthritis. *Internal Medicine,* 1988: 148: 969-70.

8. Cassell G. Infectious Causes of Chronic Inflammatory Diseases and Cancer. *Emerging Infectious Diseases* (Center for Disease Control). 1998: 4 (3).

9. Huang S, Li J, Wu J, Meng L, Shou C. Mycoplasma Infections and Different Human Carcinomas. *World Journal of Gastroenterology,* 2001:7 (2): 266-9.

10. Chen S, Tsai C, Nouri S. Carditis Associated With Mycoplasma Pneumoniae Infection. Archives: Pediatrics and Adolescent Medicine. *Am J Dis Child*, 1986: 140: 471-472.

11. Decaux G, Szyper M, Ectors M, Cornil A, Franken L. Central Nervous System Complications of Mycoplasma Pneumoniae. *Journal of Neurology, Neurosurgery and Psychiatry,* 1980: 43: 883-887.

12. Soan M, Ravnik I, Benina D, Dov P, Zakotnik B, Jazbec J. Neurological Symptoms in Patients Whose Cerebrospinal Fluid is Culture Negative and/or PCR Positive for Mycoplasma Pneumoniae. *Clinical Infectious Diseases,* 2001: 32: e31-e35.

13. Mulder L, Spierings E. Stroke in a Young Adult with Mycoplasma Pneumoniae Infection Complicated by Intravascular Coagulation. *Neurology,* 1987: 37: 1430-1431.

14. Harloff A, Voigt S, Hetzel A, Glocker F, Els T. Severe Axonal Polyradiculoneuritis and Brainstem Encephalitis Due to Mycoplasma Pneumoniae Infection. *European Jnl of Neurology,* 2002: 9: 541-545.

15. Lamaze O, Levee O, Schwarz S, Hennerici M. Mycoplasma Pneumoniae Infection as a Treatable Cause of Brainstem Encephalitis. *Neurology,* 2003: 60:1813.

16. Lam K, Bayer A. Mycoplasma Pneumoniae as a Cause of the 'Fever of Unknown Origin' Syndrome. *Internal Medicine,* 1982: 142: 2312.

17. Grüllich C, Thomas F, Baumert, Blum H. Acute Mycoplasma Pneumoniae Infection Presenting as Cholestatic Hepatitis. J*ournal of Clinical Microbiology,* 2003: 41 (1): 514–515.

18. Fernald G. Immunologic Mechanisms Suggested in the Association of Mycoplasma Pneumoniae Infection and Extrapulmonary Disease: A Review. *Yale Journal of Biology and Medicine,* 1983: 56 (5-6): 475-479.

19. Pardes Berger R, Wadowksy R. Rhabdomyolysis Associated With Infection by Mycoplasma Pneumoniae: A Case Report. *Pediatrics,* 2000: 105: 433–436.

20. Said M, Layani M, Colon S, Faraj G, Glastre C, Cochat P. Mycoplasma Pneumoniae-Associated Nephritis in Children. *Pediatric Nephrology,* 1999: 13 (1): 39-44.

21. Odom A R. Five Questions About Non-Mevalonate Isoprenoid Synthesis. *PloS Pathog.*, 2011: 7 (12): e10002323.

22. Wang et al. L-Forms of H. Pylori. *World J. Gastroenterology,* 2003: 9 (3): 525-28.

23. Blum et al. Helicobacter pylori and Probiotics. *The Journal of Nutrition*, 2007: 137: 812S-818S.

24. Chennoll et al. Novel Probiotic *Bifidobacterium bifidum* CECT 7366 Strain Active against the Pathogenic Bacterium *Helicobacter pylori. Applied and Environmental Microbiology,* 2011: 77 (4): 1335-43.

25. Wade A, Yamasaki E, Hirayama T. *Helicobacter pylori* Vacuolating Cytotoxin, VacA, Is Responsible for Gastric Ulceration. *The Journal of Biochemistry,* 2004: 136 (6): 741-46.

26. Kohda et al. Role of Apoptosis Induced by Helicobacter pylori Infection in the Development of Duodenal Ulcer. *Gut,* 1999: 44 (4): 456-62.

27. Slutter A. Infection with Chlamydia Pneumoniae in Neuronal Cells Alters the Expression of Genes Involved in Apoptosis and Autophagy Pathways. DigitalCommons@PCOM.1-1-2011.

28. Sessa et al. Chlamydia Pneumoniae Induces T cell Apoptosis Through Glutathione Redox Imbalance and Secretion of TNF-Alpha. *Int J Immunolpathol Pharmacol,* 2009: 22 (3): 659-68.

29. Byrne G, Ojcius D. Chlamydia and Apoptosis: Life and Death Decisions of an Intracellular Pathogen. *Microbiology,* 2004:2: 802-08.

30. Sokolova et al. Mycoplasma Infection Can Sensitize Host Cells to Apoptosis Through Contribution of Apoptotic-Like Endonuclease(s). *Immunol Cell Biol*, 1998: 76 (6): 526-34.

31. Zhang S, Lo SC. Effect of Mycoplasmas on Apoptosis of 32D Cells is Species-Dependent. *Curr Microbiol.*, 2007: 54 (5): 388-95.

32. Hopfe M, Henrich B. OppA, the ecto-ATPase of *Mycoplasma hominis* induces ATP release and cell death in HeLa cells. *BMC Microbiology,* 2008: 8: (55).

33. Menard et al. A Gliotoxic Factor and Amyotrophic Lateral Sclerosis. *Journal of the Neurological Sciences,* 1998: 154 (2): 209-221.

34. Lewis et al. Detection of Gliotoxin in Experimental and Human Aspergillosis. *Infect Immun.*, 2005: 73 (1): 635-37.

35. Yoseph. How Statin Drugs Really Lower Cholesterol *And Kill You One Cell at a Time.* 2012: 245-250.

36. Morrissey R E. Teratogenic Potential of the Mycotoxin, Citreoviridin, in Rats. *Fd Chem. Toxic.,* 1986: 24 (12): 1315.

37. Kiessliong Karl-Heinz. Biochemical Mechanism of Action of Mycotoxins. *Appl. Chem.*, 1986: 58(2):327-338.

38. ABC News: Statins May Cause Muscle Damage in Some Patients (2009 video).

39. Nobumasa H, Kazuo Y, Tomoko S, Harumi O, Tatsuya H, Mikako T. Elevation of Cellular NAD Levels by Nicotinic Acid and Involvement of Nicotinic Acid Phosphoribotransferase in Human Cells. J. *Biol. Chem.*, 2007: 282 (34): 24574-24582.

40. Shin M, Maeda S, Hashimoto Y, Sano K, Umezawa C. NAD Synthesis From Nicotinic Acid by the Hepatocytes Prepared From Diabetic Rats. *International Journal of Vitamin and Nutritional Research,* 1995: 65 (2): 143-6.

41. Erejuwa O et al. Glibenclamide or Metformin Combined with Honey Improves Glycemic Control in Streptozotocin-Induced Diabetic Rats. *International Journal of Biological Sciences,* 2011: 7 (2): 244-252

ALS-RELATED BOOKS BY THE YOSEPHS:

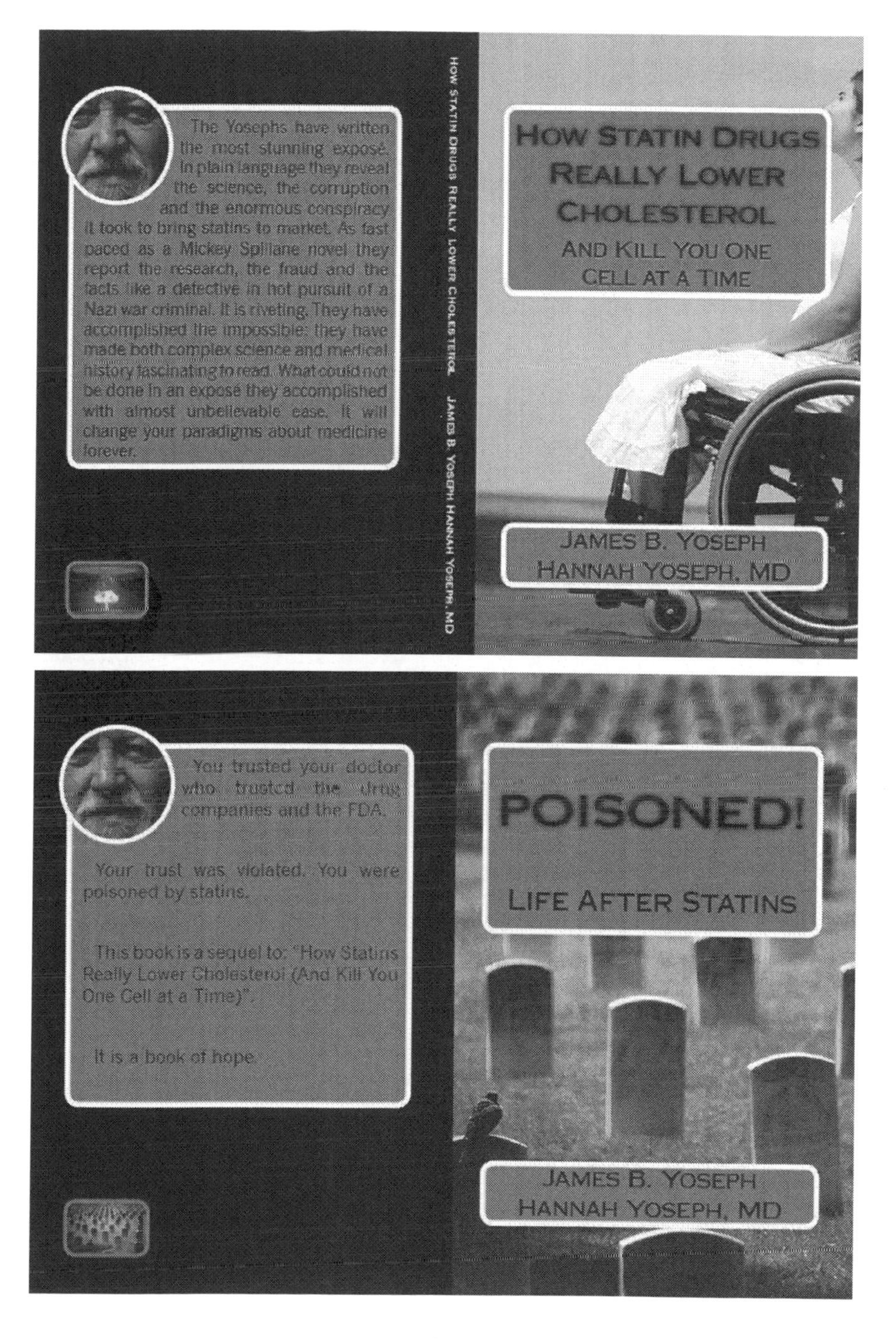